T0367559

In *Lip Service*, husband-and-wife sex experts Don and Debra Macleod show readers how they can use one of the most important sex organs (the mouth!) to spice up their love lives. Here are fresh ideas and innovative techniques for:

- Verbal seduction (aka dirty talk)
- The art of the "full-body kiss"
- The sexiest body-massage techniques known to man and woman
- And, of course, mind-blowing oral sex

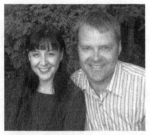

© *Darlene Vandenakerboom*

Don and Debra Macleod are the husband-and-wife authors of *Lube Jobs: A Woman's Guide to Great Maintenance Sex* and *The French Maid: And 21 More Naughty Sex Fantasies to Surprise and Arouse Your Man.*

A Woman's Guide to

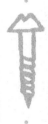

LIP SERVICE

the Art of Oral Sex and Seduction

Don and Debra Macleod

JEREMY P. TARCHER/PENGUIN

a member of Penguin Group (USA) Inc.

New York

JEREMY P. TARCHER/PENGUIN
Published by the Penguin Group
Penguin Group (USA) Inc., 375 Hudson Street, New York, New York 10014, USA • Penguin Group (Canada),
90 Eglinton Avenue East, Suite 700, Toronto, Ontario M4P 2Y3, Canada (a division of Pearson Canada Inc.) •
Penguin Books Ltd, 80 Strand, London WC2R 0RL, England • Penguin Ireland, 25 St Stephen's Green,
Dublin 2, Ireland (a division of Penguin Books Ltd) • Penguin Group (Australia), 250 Camberwell Road,
Camberwell, Victoria 3124, Australia (a division of Pearson Australia Group Pty Ltd) • Penguin Books
India Pvt Ltd, 11 Community Centre, Panchsheel Park, New Delhi–110 017, India • Penguin Group (NZ),
67 Apollo Drive, Rosedale, North Shore 0632, New Zealand (a division of Pearson New Zealand Ltd) •
Penguin Books (South Africa) (Pty) Ltd, 24 Sturdee Avenue, Rosebank, Johannesburg 2196, South Africa

Penguin Books Ltd, Registered Offices: 80 Strand, London WC2R 0RL, England

Copyright © 2009 by Don and Debra Macleod
All rights reserved. No part of this book may be reproduced, scanned, or distributed in any
printed or electronic form without permission. Please do not participate in or encourage piracy
of copyrighted materials in violation of the authors' rights. Purchase only authorized editions.
Published simultaneously in Canada

Library of Congress Cataloging-in-Publication Data

Macleod, Don.
Lip service: a his and hers guide to the art of oral sex and seduction / Don and Debra Macleod.
P.   cm.
ISBN 978-1-58542-696-6
1. Oral sex.   2. Sex instruction.   I. Macleod, Debra.   II. Title.
HQ31.5.073M33   2009   2008039067
613.9'6—dc22

BOOK DESIGN BY MEIGHAN CAVANAUGH

Neither the publisher nor the authors are engaged in rendering professional advice or services to the individual
reader. The ideas, procedures, and suggestions contained in this book are not intended as a substitute for consulting
with your physician. All matters regarding your health require medical supervision. Neither the authors nor the
publisher shall be liable or responsible for any loss or damage allegedly arising from any information or suggestion
in this book.

While the authors have made every effort to provide accurate telephone numbers and Internet addresses at the time
of publication, neither the publisher nor the authors assume any responsibility for errors, or for changes that occur
after publication. Further, the publisher does not have any control over and does not assume any responsibility for
author or third-party websites or their content.

147204767

Acknowledgments

Thank you to Joel Fotinos and Sara Carder for continuing to support our work. Thanks also to everyone at Tarcher, including Katherine Obertance for her first-rate editing, and Laura Ingman and Jennifer Levy for their publicity work.

As always, we extend our gratitude and friendship to Susan Raihofer, the literary agent of any writer's dreams. Your general brilliance and your ability to critique adult-rated proposals with such cool clarity, especially while riding the train, amaze us.

Contents

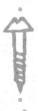

LIP SERVICE

Introduction: The Mouth as a Sexual Organ

D o a mental search of the term *female sex organ*. What image comes to mind? An academic sketch of the female body, maybe a compilation of the ones you've seen in medical textbooks with the subject pictured in a frontal anatomical stance, feet apart, arms to the side, gonads showing? Or one of those plastic, three-dimensional, genital-game-cube teaching tools, the ones where someone has lost the tiny clitoris puzzle piece? Perhaps words come to mind instead of images: *Vagina. Cervix. Ovaries. Uterus. Bartholin's glands. Fallopian tubes. Labia. Vulva.*

Mouth.

No?

That's unfair. After all, what's sexier than an alluring "I want you" smile or a tempting "take me now" pout? Flip through pages of just about any popular magazine—men's or women's—and you'll find a woman's mouth is front and center in the ads, her suggestively parted lips selling everything from cars and men's razors to perfume and movies. Sex sells, and a sexy kisser is a persuasive mouthpiece.

But it's not just big-business marketing professionals who recognize the erotic power and potential of a sexy mouth. Women know it, too. We coat our lips in sultry gloss and overpriced designer-name lipstick, soak our orthodontically straightened teeth in whitening peroxide, swish mouthwash like it's the elixir of youth, and carry mini-packets of dental floss in our handbags. Some of us even go as far as brushing our teeth in strange public washrooms. And then there's the silicone division, those who inject and inflate their lips until they look like shiny red balloon animals you're almost afraid to stand next to, lest they pop lip filler in your eyes.

Why such mouth measures? Simple. Because we instinctively realize that no other body part is as seductive, versatile, or erotically useful as a woman's mouth. Your breasts may be beautiful, but they can't fellate worth a darn. Your clitoris may be fun, but it can't give him a skin-tingling kiss on his lower back. Your pubic hair might sport a sweet heart shape, but it can't whisper sweet nothings into your lover's ear. And there aren't enough pages in this book to list all the things the Bartholin's glands can't do.

So that settles it. The mouth is an uncredited sex organ. But that doesn't mean we have to underappreciate it or, worse, underuse it; sadly many women do. Ask yourself honestly: When was the last time you used a new and exciting mouth move on your man? When was the last time he squirmed with pleasure at the feel of your lips? If you're guilty of just puckering up for a predictable suck-and-stroke blow job, it's time to update your oral skills. After all, the art of oral sex isn't just about skillful fellatio techniques; it's also about oral seduction. The more you can arouse your man before fellatio begins, the better the blow job will be.

Enter *Lip Service*, a woman's guide to using her mouth—that lip-smacking sex organ—as the ultimate seduction tool and pleasure provider. *Lip Service* will teach you how to seduce and then sexually satisfy your man in deliciously mouthwatering and (mostly) hands-free ways by learning to master the three oral arts of dirty talk, full-body kissing, and fellatio.

First, you'll learn to use the art of dirty talk to ignite your man's libido and bring him to an intense state of arousal, making his ears burn and his lust swell. Next, you'll master the art of the full-body kiss and treat him to the most exquisite, enrapturing mouth massage any man could imagine, one that will have him melting into the mattress. Finally, you'll learn to perform the fellatio of your man's fantasies by perfecting an erotic arsenal of oral sex techniques, tips, positions, and blow-job bonuses that will make his wildest wet dreams come true. Using everything from tongue twists to sex toys, you'll go from novice to expert in the time it takes him to clutch the sheets.

So lick those lips and start reading; you have some serious lip service to perform tonight. Just don't be surprised if, come dawn, your man's good-morning peck on the cheek turns into a passionate lip-lock.

1 : The Art of Dirty Talk

Now that we've agreed that the mouth is a sadly underappreciated sexual organ, let's begin exploiting its erotic potential by learning some language skills. Did you just flash back to junior high and a chalkboard scrawled with sentence fragments? If so, fear not. Our study surrounds wicked words and sexy sighs, not dangling modifiers or Latin roots.

Dirty talk is a very natural way for a woman to use her mouth to entice and excite her man during all stages and types of sexual activity. Yet despite its naturalness, many women clam up between the sheets, depriving both themselves and their partners of this aural pleasure. Why? Who knows. Perhaps we think only "sluts" use "that kind of language." Or perhaps we just don't know what to say. Whatever the reason, it's time to put our inhibitions to rest and to exercise our freedom of speech instead.

Bedtime Bawdy Talk—How to Begin

What words come to mind when you think of dirty talk? Most likely, the words you first think of are the spray-painted obscenities that grace the concrete pillars of interstate overpasses. But effective dirty talk isn't that obvious, and it needn't be that vulgar. Truly sexy speech doesn't begin by launching into a sudden verbal assault of *cock*, *pussy*, *fuck*, and so forth. Starting off with a subtle, suggestive change in tone, perhaps delivered with a sincere compliment, is a good way to ease into the art of dirty talk. A simple "You look sexy lying there like that" will suffice. The word *sexy* has an

My boyfriend is fantastic in bed, but now and then he'll say something dirty that misses the mark. Sometimes it almost makes me laugh. How can I tell him without hurting his feelings?

♂ *Don*: If he only misses the mark "now and then," let it go. The male ego is fragile. Try beating him to the punch by telling him, in the heat of things, what you want him to say to you. That's a sexy time to teach him what to say.

♀ *Debra*: Focus on the positive. Instead of saying "I don't like it when you say X," try saying "I love it when you say Y." And when he does hit the mark, react strongly so he can see which words have an effect on you and which don't.

alluring quality that always has a wonderful effect. Who doesn't like to hear that someone finds them sexy?

When you climb into bed, reach for your man and give him a long, deep kiss on the mouth to arouse him. As he responds, voice a low moan of pleasure and eagerly press your body into him to show him how fast he's turning you on. Remember the role that body language plays in communication: It's as important in the bedroom as anywhere else, so be very aware of it at all times. Unwavering eye contact communicates desperate want. Keep your eyes fixed on his, only tearing them away to eagerly admire his body. Draw your eyes down his arms, his chest, and ever downward. If he's wearing pajamas or underwear, smile hungrily and take them off without waiting for his permission.

As his nakedness is revealed, break into a wide mischievous grin. Tell him how good he looks and how seeing his bare body makes you feel. You can say something like "Sweetie, you look wonderful. You turn me on so much. I've been waiting all day to see you naked like this."

Keep it simple and sincere. Drag your fingers along his bare skin and continue to comment on the effect his body has on you: "Your skin feels so good, so hot under my fingers." Let a throaty groan escape your lips: "*Mmm*. I want you so much tonight."

In a bold gesture, remove your clothing and let him admire your nakedness. Don't forget body language: Move your hips to show your arousal and run your hands over your body to demonstrate your desire. Knead your breasts and pinch your nipples, biting your lower lip to betray the power of that sensation. Tell him you've been waiting all day to feel his hands on you: "I've been waiting to feel your hands on my body, your fingers touching and pinching my nipples like this."

Take your man's hands and pull them to your body. Ask him to touch you the way you've been waiting for him to: "Please touch me. I want to feel your hands moving all over me."

When your man obeys, react with obvious pleasure by writhing and moaning. Put your hands on his as he caresses you, perhaps directing him to the places you'd like to be touched. A simple "Touch me here" or "Kiss me here, yes, that feels amazing" does wonders.

While your man is caressing your body, reach out to caress his. Whenever he touches or kisses you in a way that pleasures you, react with a gasp and kiss or fondle him with more urgency. Cup his testicles and sigh, making sure to compliment them: "They're so heavy, so big... You're ready, aren't you?"

As he hardens, squeeze the shaft of his penis, then smile with eager anticipation and say something like: "You're so hard and thick, I love the way your hardness feels and tastes on my tongue. I can't wait to feel it push past my lips into my mouth and then slide down my throat."

The precise words and phrases you use aren't important; the ones we include in this chapter are merely illustrative. As long as your language is descriptive—and reflects what you're truly feeling or desiring—you'll get your point across, and the results will be stellar. In fact, you'll notice that the preceding scenario didn't feature a single official dirty word. (We're saving that for later!) Overtly lewd language isn't always necessary. In fact, depending on the atmosphere of your lovemaking and/or your personal sensibilities, it can be both distracting and artificial. Recall that dirty talk isn't about gushing out a stream of obscene words. It's about seducing your man and intensifying his sexual arousal before and during fellatio.

> The precise words you use aren't important. As long as your words are descriptive and reflect what you feel or desire, you'll make a sexy statement.

That being said, don't be afraid to test the dirty waters beyond oral sex. Although *Lip Service* uses the art of dirty talk to enhance the anticipation and pleasure of fellatio, seductive speech is nonetheless an effective way to add erotic excitement to any form of sexual activity, including hand jobs and intercourse. It's a skill that, when mastered, can find expression in many ways.

Supersized Sex—The Sound Track

"It was a fifty-eight-inch plasma big-screen, high definition," boasts Joel. "The best television money could buy. Anita bought it for me for my thirtieth birthday. I loved it."

What Joel also loved about his big-screen birthday present was his wife's promise to watch an adult film with him on it: "We were excited about it," smiles Anita. "We were curious to see what a porn would look like on such a big television." So the couple turned off the lights and curled up on the couch in front of the enormous screen, ready for the XXX premier. Joel pressed Play.

"It was a shocker," he admits. "The guy looked like he was fifty inches. He was getting blow jobs from two women. It was weird to see it all happening so . . . large."

"It was disturbing," laughs Anita. "We just stared at the screen like a couple of deer caught in the headlights. We were stunned. It did nothing to turn us on; in fact, it was a turnoff. The women were giving the man oral sex, but they kept, well, spitting on his erection for lubrication. That's *not* something you want to see supersized."

"Watching blow jobs usually turns me on," says Joel. "That didn't."

"We tried to get into it," Anita continues, "but we ended up moving onto the floor and spinning around to avoid looking at the screen."

But if the visual was so unappealing, why didn't they just turn off the television?

"I was going to turn it off," says Anita, "but the sound track was worth the price of admission. The sights didn't do it for us, but the actors kept saying the dirtiest things and making really arousing sounds. Most porns we've watched are heavy on the visuals and the sounds are kind of secondary, but this one was different. There was lots of dirty talk, and it was a real turn-on."

"We ended up turning up the volume and having sex to the sound track," Joel recalls. "It was intense, especially since Anita never talked dirty and I wasn't used to hearing it. I couldn't believe it when she started to whisper a few of the things the actors were saying."

"That was an eye-opening experience," adds Anita, "in more than one way. I could tell the language was making Joel more frantic, and his orgasm was really strong. Mine was, too. I guess the movie turned out to be educational ... I learned my partner liked to hear dirty talk, and I learned that I liked hearing and saying it, too."

The surprise dirty talk might've been fun for Joel and Anita in the heat of the moment, but was it just a passing novelty, or did it last?

"We don't use it every time we have sex," Anita continues, "but it's definitely a regular visitor in our bedroom now."

And how does Anita's speech-giving measure up to the pros?

"Anita's dirty talk isn't always as colorful as that of the porn stars," says Joel. "That's probably a good thing. I find the *way* she says something is more arousing than the particular words she uses. She's got quite the mouth on her—I mean that in a good way!"

"There are lots of words I won't say," Anita echoes, "but I always make sure I speak in a sexy way. It makes me feel more sensual, and it works wonders on Joel's libido."

Now that dirty talk is a regular part of their sex life, does Anita ever feel the need to expand her vocabulary to keep her erotic edge?

"Sometimes I feel like I'm saying the same things over and over, kind of like I'm stuck in a dirty-talk rut," says Anita. "When that happens I'll ask Joel to get a porn, and I'll listen to the things the women say. I'll usually pick up one or two new phrases that I hadn't thought of."

But what about the big-screen? Is it still host to adult-movie night?

"We don't watch porn on the big-screen anymore," Joel reveals. "Sometimes what you don't see is more exciting than what you do see."

"Maybe that's the draw of erotic language," reasons Anita. "It engages senses that many couples don't usually use. People watch adult movies, touch each other, experiment with toys and positions but don't always take advantage of the simplest things—like their own voices and sexual imagination. Dirty talk lets you do that."

Finally, how has "dirty talk" changed this couple's love life?

"Fantasies," says Joel. "We never used to, but now we feel very free to talk about and explore our sexual fantasies in bed. It's very liberating and very exciting."

"That's true," Anita adds. "Once you get used to speaking to each other in a more sexual way, you find that your sex life opens up in other ways, too. Our sexual communication is far easier and more honest than it used to be. That's been our experience, anyway. I think that as long as you don't compromise yourself by saying things you're not comfortable with, dirty talk can be good, clean fun."

Lost for Words

Many women who haven't used dirty talk in their sex lives cite not knowing what to say as the main reason they haven't used this erotic tool. Anita used pornographic movies to expand her erotic vocabulary. Other women may prefer erotica, including online erotic stories or "harder" romance novels. But here's a simple tip that might help: Focus on what you're doing and feeling—or on what you're going to do—rather than on word choice, particularly in the early seduction phase. Think of yourself as a sexcaster and describe the play as it happens.

If you're kissing your man's neck, whisper something in his ear, like:

 Don't know the lingo? Think of yourself as a sexcaster and describe the play as it happens.

- You smell so good, so sexy.
- I love this part of your body, but I can't wait to move down.
- Your neck and shoulders are so strong, I love kissing them.

If you're kissing his chest or stomach, you can say:
- Your skin tastes wonderful.
- Your chest feels so powerful.
- I want to move down your body; I want to taste more of you.

As you move down his body to lick his thighs, try saying:
- I can feel your hardness brushing against my face.
- I'm so close to your thickness, I can't wait to feel it in my mouth.
- You smell so good, I know you'll taste even better.

And always remember to communicate your own desire:
- I love feeling your nakedness against mine.
- Kissing your skin makes me ache between my legs.
- Your body is so sexy, it turns me on so much.

If you wish, you can bring your partner into the carnal conversation. Many men love to say dirty things as much as they like to hear them, so see if your man is one of them. You can start by simply asking him how he feels when you touch him:

- Does it feel good when I kiss you here?
- How does this feel?
- Does it make you hard when I lick you like this?

Or ask him what he wants you to do:

- Do you want me to keep doing this?
- Are you ready for me to suck you?
- Do you want me to lick or suck your balls?

You can also ask him how your body feels to him:

- Can you feel how tight my nipples are?
- Can you feel how wet I'm getting for you?
- Run your hands over my skin...Can you feel my goose bumps from your touch?

As your man's desire builds and his physical needs grow, make sure that your dirty talk keeps pace with what's happening. When you're ready to perform oral sex, tell him you can't wait any longer to have him in your mouth. Moan eagerly as you push your lips onto his penis, thereby compounding his physical pleasure with the erotic sound of your desire. Some men feel pleasurable vibrations on their penis if a woman "hums" a long, low *Mmm* while she has it in her mouth.

Now and then, take a strategic break from your mouth maneuvers for some well-spoken dirty talk:

- Your shaft feels so hard and smooth against my lips.
- The tip is so swollen, so sensitive.
- I love licking your whole length...It's so big, so powerful.

Okay, get ready. It's time to say the kind of things he *really*

wants to hear. Stop sucking, and try something more explicit, perhaps something along the lines of:

- I want to suck the juice out of you...I need to feel it slide
  down my throat.
- Grab my hair and thrust harder, fuck my mouth like you
  would fuck my pussy.
- Slide your cock over my tongue, explode on it; I want to
  swallow your milk.

The practice of "deep throating" is exciting to many men,
so go ahead and make reference to it as he begins to thrust with
more intensity, even if you can't perform it. The idea of being deep-
throated may be enough to flare the mental aspect of his growing
orgasm, and you can bring him to the threshold of climax by looking him in the eyes and saying:

- I love to feel your cock rocketing down my throat; it makes
  my clit throb.
- Pump your dick past my lips...faster, harder...Let the
  come pool in your balls.
- Fuck my mouth/throat deeper, it feels incredible...You're
  close; let it go now.

More graphic or "vulgar" language will also do the trick, but
only you can decide what words you're willing to use and what
erotic ambience you want to set with your partner, whether you
and he are engaging in oral sex or another form of sexual activity.

You're the sole judge of what words and phrases you're comfortable with, as well as what type of language you think your partner will respond to. Dirty talk is a subjective game, and every couple must make their own rules.

For example, the "C" word won't appear in this chapter. That doesn't mean it can't be effective, but it must be said by a woman who is comfortable saying it and be heard by a man who will like hearing it. Debra won't say that word, and Don doesn't miss it in the lineup. You might feel differently. The dirty words and erotic lines suggested here are just that—suggestions—and they're not as graphic as others you've heard or may prefer. Your comfort level ultimately determines your word choice. An out-of-place or out-of-character word can both sabotage your sexy speech and make you feel unnecessarily self-conscious. Keep it authentic, and you can't go wrong.

 While dirty talk should be spontaneous and un-scripted, new speakers may find it helpful to choose their words and phrases in advance.

Dirty talk should be as spontaneous as possible. For the uninitiated and unpracticed, however, it is helpful to have an idea in advance of what you're going to say. We hope the words and phrases we've included in this chapter will be of use. The words *cock*, *pussy*, and *fuck* are almost essential entry-level dirty words that obviously have more sexual appeal than such clinical terms as *penis*, *vagina*, or *coitus*. Adding descriptive elements to these basic dirty words adds to their flexibility and effect, and is an easy way to increase your bedroom vocabulary.

For example, you can compliment your man on his *hard, thick cock* and tell him that your *wet, swollen pussy* wants to feel it as much as your *hot, hungry mouth* wants to taste it. A purred *Fuck my mouth slowly* followed by a rabid *Fuck my throat deeper, faster*, are instructions he won't have any problem following. It may not be poetry, but it'll have him swooning all the same.

As a general rule, it's a good idea to use dirty words in short sentences or expressions of pleasure. It's also best to avoid overloading your speech with strong words, à la *My pussy wants to fuck your fucking cock* or *Shove your fucking dick down my fucking throat*. Using more than one or two spicy words in a sentence may overcook the dish. Keep it short and sweet. You're not reciting some gutter version of an epic Greek poem, you're just trying to show your man how aroused you are and, in the process, to increase his arousal as well.

Mood Music

We've all experienced it at the movies—that swell of sentimental music that accompanies the heroine's words of undying love and makes both her lover and the audience believe in her sincerity. Or that long, tense, disturbing tone that makes us hold our breath and dread the moment we know is coming: the moment when whatever evil has been lurking behind the closed door is about to pounce on the bra-and-panty–clad victim. Background sounds and music can enhance, sometimes even set, the mood in the movies. In the same way, the sounds you make and the tone of your voice can work with the words you speak to increase the eroticism of your dirty talk. Think of your tone and sounds—your moans, groans, grunts, and sighs—as mood music to accompany your sexy script.

As you're talking dirty, be conscious of the tone of your voice and remember that it, as well as the sounds you make, depends on what sexual stage you're at. During seduction, keep your voice low and throaty, with slow, deep moans. But as your sex session intensifies, so, too, should your voice. You should speak louder and more desperately, with ecstatic moans and long-lasting groans.

The mood music you choose also depends on the type of sex and sexual release you and your lover are engaging in. For example, soft sighs and whispered words are perfect for slow, face-to-face intercourse and mutual orgasm, while nasty, hard grunts and groans complement frenzied from-behind penetration and selfish satisfaction. Muttered moans and long, agonized murmurs are very effective during slow-paced oral sex, while short, frantic gasps suit faster-paced fellatio.

Voice tone can also change the way words or phrases sound. A whispered *I love the way you fuck me* during sweet lovemaking conveys a different sense than a shouted *Fuck me harder* during a sinful quickie. Therefore, choose the mood you want to set, and then choose your words, tone, and sounds accordingly.

"Rough-and-Tumble" Talk

Chances are, your proficiency in the art of dirty talk will have a powerful effect on your man and will make him more eager than usual. Allowing oral sex to get a little "rough" (all in fun, of course) will let him get the most out of his lustful burst of libido. Some men are very turned on by the idea of actively thrusting into a woman's mouth rather than just being passively sucked. Why not play along and let your partner let loose a bit?

Just remember that how eager your partner gets is entirely up to you and that regardless of the erotic impression you're giving him, you should always be in control when performing fellatio. If he isn't the type to stick to your rules, skip this part of the game.

You can also use your body language to ramp the voracity of your man's arousal by clutching his hips as though encouraging him to thrust faster or deeper into your mouth. Putting his hands on your head so that he can direct your mouth is similarly effective, as is licking your lips hungrily before taking him in your mouth. You can plead with him to *Go faster, harder* and—if you want to really push him to the edge—*Slam your cock down my throat*. It may be nasty, but in the heat of a rough-and-tumble oral sex session, it's irresistibly erotic.

Give your man permission to say whatever he wants to you, and don't be shocked if he says something you wouldn't have expected. Dirty sex rouses dirty thoughts, which in turn result in dirty words. It's not uncommon for normally conservative men to call their wives a "slut" or "whore" or "bitch" during raunchy oral sex or rough intercourse. Unless you're strongly opposed, why not indulge him and let him escape into the moment? Chances are, you'll be sharing a laugh about it inside of five minutes. So long as he's loving and respectful to you in your relationship, let him enjoy slandering you in bed once in a while.

Reaching the Finish Line

Keep in mind that dirty talk—including word choice, voice tone and sounds, and body language—doesn't lose importance as your man reaches orgasm. What athlete slows down as he nears the finish line? Don't lose momentum or greet your man's moment of glory with silence. Instead, react loudly and squirm like your body is absorbing his burst of pleasure. Your reaction to his orgasm can both prolong and amplify his enjoyment.

When you know he's near climax, smile eagerly before going down for the count, and say something like:

- You're so close, your balls are tight and ready to explode.
- I can feel the veins on your cock throbbing.
- I can't wait to swallow it all.

This kind of dirty talk heightens anticipation and lets your man revel in the exquisite pleasure of his orgasm's peak. The more intense that peak is the more incredible the release will be. A well-timed *You're making me come, too!* may also add intensity to the mental element of his impending climax (whether it's true or not).

As your man ejaculates, grip his penis tightly with your lips. Gasp, moan, or even squeal with blissful abandon as he comes in your mouth. Breathless, pained sounds of sexual pleasure groaned against his groin as he climaxes will be filthy music to his ears. Just be sure to keep your mouth on him and maintain your rhythm and pressure until he's finished—sexy throat sounds will have to suffice.

Finally, as his orgasm subsides, keep stroking him with your hands until his pleasure is exhausted. You can prolong the happy memory by showering him with compliments, such as:

- You came so hard.
- There was so much of it... It tasted so good.
- I love to feel it warm and thick in my mouth.

Whatever words or description you use, make sure your man knows how much you enjoyed the feel of his orgasm. Most men will appreciate a dirty compliment!

Carnal Keystrokes

If any proof of a man's desire for dirty talk were required, one need only go online and scroll through the staggering number of sex "chat rooms" that are open for business. Cybersex is a phenomenally popular activity that attracts millions of men both around the world and around the clock, and its popularity seems only to be growing. Wearing nothing more than a user I.D. and password, many men can now scratch their dirty talk itches in the privacy of their own computer screen.

Here's a toned-down sampling of what you might read:

Hard4U: >> I spread your legs wide and put the head of my rock-hard cock against your pussy...you're so ready and tight.
Clean&Shaved: >> Oh drive it in deep, I'm ready to come...slide it past my clit...aaaahhh!

Hard4U: >> Yeah, take it all, all ten inches, you whore.

Clean&Shaved: >> Aaaahhh...Oh God that was good...was it good for you?

Hard4U: >> Hard4U is now offline.

I found some printouts of my husband's cybersex activity. He's been having conversations with somebody called tightnbare. When I confronted him, he said he was doing it because I won't talk dirty. Should I start? I tried it, but I hate it.

♀ *Debra:* When it comes to sex, you should never do anything you "hate." You'll just feel compromised and resentful. I'd add that secret online sex chat is a bad idea in a monogamous relationship. Alternatives might be dirty stories from the net, reading other people's sex chat together, or buying a book of published erotica or pornographic writing.

♂ *Don:* Nothing is better than getting a surprise flirty e-mail from Deb and firing one back. YOU should be his online sex partner. Maybe you'll find it easier to type the words than to say them. Your husband should be satisfied with that. If he isn't, he's online for another reason.

No, it isn't the most sophisticated piece of literature you'll ever read, but for many people, it satisfies a craving. The fact is, cybersex is becoming ever more common as both men and women get turned on, and sometimes even addicted, to its allure. The sexual effect of seeing obscene, lewdly descriptive words on the screen, particularly when those words are directed at the reader, is powerful. Toss in the anonymity and the rose-colored hue of imagination, and the fantasy is complete. (No, of course I'm not a flabby, forty-year-old comic-book store manager living in my mom's basement; I'm a 6'2", 200-pound professional with a muscular build.)

Please Hold While I Transfer Your Call

Yet even as the World Wide Web makes free virtual sex a reality for millions, its more vocal and costly cousin—phone sex—is still on the line and holding strong. Even today, there is an abundance of phone sex/chat lines that operate 24/7, filling credit-card-holding men's ears with taboo fantasies, deep-throated *ooh*'s and *ahh*'s, and unscripted sex talk. It's more than sexy; it's financially savvy. And phone sex has a definite advantage over the cold *click click click* of the keyboard. It offers the caller immediate interaction, freedom from having to hit Send during an inopportune moment, and the excitement of hearing a real woman's voice in real time. There's nothing like the classics.

But is there anything the good girl can learn from the bad girl on the other end of the phone-sex line? After all, they're the pros. If anyone can offer advice on using the mouth as a sexual organ, it's these velvet-voiced operators.

So, in the line of duty, we called one up. After approximately forty dollars' worth of explaining ourselves—we're sex writers wanting to ask some questions, not customers wanting to chat—we enjoyed a surprisingly fascinating conversation with Jessica, a spirited phone-sex operator with three years' experience.

> Dirty talk is a necessary sex skill, one that women need to
> have; otherwise, their men just call me.
>
> —*Jessica, Phone-Sex Operator*

"I get lots of customers who are in relationships, but whose wives or girlfriends won't say the kinds of things that really turn them on," says Jessica. "These are normal enough guys, they just want to hear something more exciting than "Oh yeah" or "Are you done?" so they phone somebody like me before going to bed with their girl. They're my best calls because they're polite and they're not cheap. But I also get a lot of customers who want it all laid out, the uglier the better. They get off on hearing a string of dirty words—it doesn't matter if I sound like I'm into it or not—and when they talk, it's almost always hard-core. Totally impersonal, those guys wouldn't care if I was a recording. And they usually hang up before they come, just to save a buck."

What kinds of things do they say, you ask? Well, we asked, too.

"Lots of talk about oral sex; it's number one," reveals Jessica. "It's rare that I'm surprised by what a guy says anymore. It's never very imaginative, just variations of the usual smut talk. 'Suck my cock 'til you gag, I want to drive my tongue up your ass, can you bite your own tits, I've got a hard-on that could split you open,' that kind of thing," says Jessica, adding, "And lots of grunting and slapping noises that get louder the more excited they get."

Anything bordering on . . . romantic?

Jessica laughs a little too long and then pauses in thought before offering an amused reply. "I wouldn't call it *romantic*, but some do get more satisfaction out of hearing an erotic story or fantasy, or hearing me masturbate while they talk. Those are the ones who tend to play along more: I say something, and they give something back. There's a back-and-forth that they really like. I have a lot of repeat customers who are like that."

And what kind of relationship does Jessica have with her repeat customers?

"I know personal stuff about many of my repeat guys," she reveals. "We spend time in small talk so they can get comfortable talking to me and come out of their shell. Many repeats want to feel like they know me and that I know them on a more personal level. I guess they find it sexier if somebody they know is talking dirty to them instead of a stranger." Another laugh. "That's about as romantic as it gets."

Does Jessica have any thoughts about why "normal" men in monogamous relationships would want phone sex?

"Some men have things they want to hear somebody say, lots of stuff they want to say, but they can't say it when they're in bed with their wife or girlfriend. Maybe they're scared she's going to think they're perverted. But when they're talking to me, anything goes, and they can explore that side of their sexuality. Sometimes a guy won't want to have an orgasm while he's on the phone; he'll just want me to get him hot, then he'll go jump into bed with his woman and let it out. If that doesn't say he isn't getting what he wants, I don't know what does. That's why I say women need to talk dirty. Guys get off on it; there's no way around it."

Finally, does Jessica—phone-sex operator extraordinaire—have any advice for women who are new to the racy realm of dirty talk?

"Lighten up," Jessica says. "Start slow and build your confidence. It really helps if you can get into it. There are some customers who really turn me on, and I'll sometimes use that arousal all night to make my calls better. It's way easier to talk dirty to somebody else if you're turned on yourself. I'd also tell women to practice. When I started, I didn't know what to say. Some words would get stuck in my throat because I wasn't used to saying them. You can always get some erotic stories and dirty words to practice reading out loud. That's what I did, and it got a lot easier."

Overall, a worthwhile conversation, even *after* we received our credit card statement.

There are two particularly valuable things we can take from Jessica's insight. First, that many men are neither hearing nor saying what they want in bed. Some men call Jessica, some visit chat rooms, and some just go without. Is there a chance your man could be aroused by more explicit language or word imagery, particularly during fellatio? Is there a chance *you* could be aroused by it, too? You won't know until you try. Add a few well-timed nasty words to your sexual vocabulary, and see the results.

Practice Makes Perfect

The second important thing we learned from Jessica is that reading erotic stories aloud is a useful way for a woman to practice vocalizing dirty words. Accordingly, we've included a short erotic story for you to practice reciting. Read the story aloud as many times as necessary to feel at ease with it. If it becomes elementary, try injecting a few colorful adjectives or ideas of your own, thereby

Is it true that men like "screamers"? I honestly don't know if it's a cliché or if it's for real.

♀ *Debra:* I think that most guys do like a more vocal sex partner. Don't you? Screaming might be over the top, but it's nice to know your lover is turned on by you.

♂ *Don:* Yes, guys love vocal sex partners. As for screaming, I don't think it's over the top, especially if you're really going at it. What man wouldn't want to be evicted from his apartment for that?

using this story as a starting point to find and then to fine-tune your own salacious speaking style.

But remember that this process isn't about forcing yourself to say dirty words; it's about finding an erotic rhythm to your speech and learning to speak in a sexually compelling way. Pace is also important, and you should note how it is used in the story. The introductory paragraphs draw readers in and seduce them. As the story proceeds and the sexual tension between the characters intensifies, so, too, does the eroticism of the language used. By the time the story climaxes, word choice is at its dirtiest peak.

The way you arouse your man in bed follows a similar pattern: You start with flirtatious words, move into more seductive phrases, and then climax with graphic word imagery. If you try to follow this model, you may be surprised at how few "obscenities" it really takes to deliver some first-class dirty talk before and during fellatio.

Another option is to snuggle under the sheets with your man and read this erotic scenario aloud to him, word for word. Tell him to close his eyes and listen to the ultimate man-friendly bedtime story, narrated by his own sexy storyteller. Just be sure to take an intermission or two to serve up some oral sex.

Regardless of whether your lascivious language is spontaneous or scripted, it'll have your man's ears burning and his lust aflame. Dirty talk is one of the sexiest ways that you can use your mouth as a sexual organ and perform some great lip service—without even smearing your lipstick.

Reading erotica out loud is a great way for a woman to practice saying dirty words and speaking in a sexual way.

The Hitchhiker

It's almost one o'clock in the morning, and you've been driving for hours. You're alone in the car with only a selection of old CDs to keep you company. There are miles of highway behind and before you, and sleep is never more than a blink away. You'd call someone on your cell phone, but it's too late. You pass a hitchhiker walking on the side of the road and watch him disappear in your rearview mirror. Maybe you should've picked him up. He'd be someone to talk to, and that would keep you alert.

A few miles later, you pass another hitchhiker. This one is a woman carrying a large red backpack. You glance in your rearview mirror and watch her until she's out of sight, your mind already wandering. You wonder what she'd look like up close, how friendly she might've been, how grateful for the ride. Fantasies start running through your mind, thoughts about pulling the car over and doing things with her. Your groin stirs and starts to ache. It's painful, but at least it's keeping you awake. You look forward to getting home and crawling into bed. You can almost feel the rough skin of your hand against the smoothness of your shaft, stroking you to release. It's going to be strong.

Another hitchhiker is up ahead, another woman carrying a large dark backpack. Perfect timing. Some small talk, even with a stranger, will keep your mind from wandering and your eyes from closing. You lay your jacket over your lap to cover your hard-on and pull over. The woman runs up to the car and smiles through the passenger-side window. She's quite pretty, athletic-looking, with slightly rosy cheeks from the warm wind. You tell yourself to keep your thoughts pure and just enjoy the company.

But as the woman opens the door and sits beside you, you quickly get the sense she isn't entirely innocent, either. She gives you a mischievous grin and closes the door, then pulls a rubber band out of her messy ponytail, letting her blonde hair fall on her shoulders. The two of you exchange introductions as you start driving. Her car ran out of gas a mile or so back, she embarrassedly admits. She's been very distracted tonight and isn't making the best judgments. You ask why, and she tells you that she's been looking forward to meeting someone tonight at Pheasant Grove Park, and the anticipation is overwhelming.

She's baiting you to ask more, you can tell, but you resist. You tell her you're driving past the park, so you can take her right there. She thanks you, then bites her lip and stares at you with devilish eyes. Your legs involuntarily twitch, and you feel your groin stir. The jacket is still on your lap, but your erection is threatening to bulge up. "Don't you want to know why I'm going to the park?" She teases. You nod with feigned indifference. "I'm part of a club," she says, "and new members are always welcome." You ask what kind of club, and she smiles before softly chastising you. "I think you know what kind of club," she flirts. "We meet online first, then we meet in person at the park. Do you like to watch or be watched?"

The woman's boldness sends a hammer of pleasure to your cock, and you shift in your seat. She notices. "It's an addiction," she continues. "Sex like that is incredible. Fucking a stranger while more strangers look on, it's a rush." Her explicit words make you harder, and you feel your balls tighten as images of her lying on the backseat, her legs open and inviting, race through your mind. You can almost feel the warmth of her flesh as your body lowers onto hers, into hers, to start pumping. You can almost feel her tightness around your shaft. Your hands grip the steering wheel, and the woman laughs.

The heavily wooded park is dark when you enter. There are at least twenty cars parked along the tree line, most with their head-lights off but interior lights on. You can see silhouettes standing outside some of the cars, and through the glass you catch glimpses of bare flesh moving within. You squirm in your seat. Even the light weight of your jacket on your groin is too pleasurable, and your cock pounds at the passing sight of a naked woman bent over the hood of a car. A man is fucking her from behind. His hands are gripping her hips and pulling her ass back against him. Her breasts are flattened against the car, and her whole body jerks forward when the man thrusts.

The woman beside you moans at the sight. "*Mmm*, that's nice," she purrs as she turns to smile invitingly at you. "Here's fine." You pull over, keeping your hands on the steering wheel and your eyes straight ahead. She opens her door but doesn't get out. You feel your jacket being pulled away, and the friction makes your cock ache. You suppress a groan. "Why hide that hard-on all the way home," the woman asks, "when I can take care of it right now?" You take a breath as you feel her hand rest on top of your throbbing bulge. She squeezes your shaft right through your jeans, then releases it to squeeze your heavy balls, holding them in her grip. You gasp. "Tell me you don't want to fuck," she dares.

The woman's body brushes against you as she reaches over to turn off the headlights. She reaches up to switch on the interior light, and you turn to look at her breasts near your face. Without another word, the woman pulls off her jacket and lifts her shirt over her head. She's wearing a white lace bra that unfastens in the front, and, before you have time to think, she undoes it to expose her full breasts, the nipples pink and taut. Your heart pounds, and so does your cock and balls. Wanting to bring you to the point of surrender, she cups her breasts and moves them in small circles, then pinches her nipples with her fingers. You lose your breath as she bends her head down and flicks her tongue over a nipple.

You can smell her sweet sweat as she brings a breast to your mouth and touches your lips with an erect nipple. You part your lips, and she puts the hard bud inside your mouth. It tastes like salty flesh, and the soft mound of her breast pressing into your nose smells like desire. You suck her tit, feeling the nipple lengthen and harden in your mouth, and she drops her head back on her shoulders. You suck it stronger, and she groans, moving her hand down to your lap. Your cock swells and throbs in agony against the restriction of your jeans. Knowing you've surrendered, the woman unzips your pants and you feel the release of fabric as your rigid thickness springs up.

Her hands are around it. You hear your own moans fill the car's interior. Her nipple is still in your mouth, and her hand is wrapped around your shaft, squeezing, pulsing. "Now," she whispers desperately. She sits back and struggles to remove her clothes while you do the same. As you undress, something catches your attention: movement outside the car's window. People are watching. Their hands are down their pants as they stare hungrily at you and the woman, waiting for you to do more with her. The reality of it hits you hard, and your dick aches from the perverse pleasure. You want to show them more. The woman was right; this is incredible.

The woman climbs into the backseat and lies down, spreading her legs wide. You follow her. Even in the low light you can see her pussy looks delicious. Your cock is standing out straight from your body, and you reach out to scoop her pussy with your hand, slipping two fingers inside. She rocks against your hand, desperate for more. She starts fucking your hand. Breathless, you look down at this woman as she gyrates her hips on the seat, squeezing her pussy around your fingers and urging you to sink them in deeper. Her clit is swollen and slippery, and her body shudders each time your thumb glides over it. You look up at the people staring in. Their hands are moving faster under their pants.

The woman spreads her legs even wider and holds them open, begging you to finish her off. You push your fingers in deeper and explore inside her, looking for her G-spot. Her back arches, and she cries out. Her pussy contracts around your fingers as the orgasm flows through her body. As she recovers and stares hotly up at you, you realize you've been stroking your shaft the whole time. She looks at it and says, "I want to suck it now. I like to feel hardness in my mouth while I'm still raw from coming."

You kneel on the seat, your naked back pressed against the cool car door. You sense someone just outside the window, only inches away from you and the woman, and you're filled with a powerful need for exhibitionism. The girl lies on her stomach and in an instant you feel her powerful suck pull your cock deep inside her mouth, down her throat. You've never been deep-throated this far before. The raw skin on the head of your cock rubs against the back of her throat. You start to pump. She moans, and the sound vibrates up your shaft, pinching it and your balls pleasurably. You pump faster. The come pools in your balls and you clench your teeth, feeling the orgasm build as her lips stroke your shaft.

You put your hands on the woman's head and push it into your groin, driving your cock into her mouth. You're almost at the peak when the woman takes her mouth off of you and sits up. Pushing you to the side, she squirms past you to open the door and step outside. Pained, you cup your balls and follow her. You sense people moving back, hiding in the trees, but you don't care. Let them watch. You want them to see what you're going to do to this woman. She walks to the front of the car and lifts herself onto the hood, lying back to stretch out her body in wait for you. You stand in front of her, staring at her full breasts and hard tits, her glistening well-groomed pussy, and her smooth legs. You're going to fuck her again, and this time you're going to finish.

Climbing onto the hood, you drop your body down onto her. No more teasing, no more showing off. Now you just want release. As your weight pins her down, she bites your ear and whispers, "Bury it in me now, in one stroke." Panting, you aim your dick between her spread legs. With a grunt, you push the head of your cock past the tight lips of her pussy, feeling your solid length sink into her. She writhes under you. "Pull it out so I can watch it again," she says. "I love to watch a cock bury itself in my pussy." You withdraw and glance toward the trees. In the darkness, you can see that a man has his hand down the pants of a woman. You stare at them as you slide your thickness back into her body.

You thrust into her again and again, feeling every inch of her smooth, hot flesh. The mounds of her breasts feel exquisite under your chest, with the hard nipples rubbing against your body. As you stroke her pussy, in and out, you feel her wet pubic hair on your cock and balls. She cries out and a gush of liquid tells you she's had another orgasm. Her pussy contracts around your shaft. You pull it out, then squeeze it past her slick lips again. And again.

You feel your balls lift and tighten, ready to explode. And then it comes. Your orgasm mounts, peaks quickly, and then hot pleasure sears your cock as wave after wave of come spills out to fill her box. It feels like liquid fire jetting out of your body, the pain and the pleasure almost inseparable. Your orgasm lasts a long time, longer than you imagined was possible, and, as it wracks your body, you look toward the trees. People are fucking. Women are on their hands and knees, being impaled from behind by grunting men. Men are lying down, with women straddling them, lowering their tight pussies onto eagerly waiting cocks.

Finally, your orgasm begins to subside. The sensation lasts, though, and you keep pumping until every drop is out of you. And the woman doesn't stop you, she wants every bit. You collapse on top of her, and the two of you, gasping for air, breathe together.

With a tired, happy sigh, the woman pushes you off and darts back into the car. She collects her clothes, dresses quickly, and throws her backpack over her shoulder. You lie back on the cool metal of the car's hood, all traces of modesty gone. The woman walks past you, offering nothing more than a sly smile and a wave good-bye as she disappears into the trees. You stumble back into your car and look at your watch.

It's almost three o'clock in the morning, but you're energized and awake enough to drive cross-country now.

2 : Male Erogenous Zones

Ask your man where his erogenous zones are, and you're likely to receive a proud "front and center" gesture, probably followed by a proposition. Sigh. They're such simple creatures, aren't they? The truth is, men actually can feel pleasure in places where the sun does shine as well as where it doesn't (or shouldn't). The arts of full-body kissing and fellatio are exquisitely pleasurable to a man, but before a woman can reach such hot destinations, she must first study the "male map" and learn the way to that greatest of all states: the state of arousal.

Body and Mind

As most of us recognize, there are two roads to arousal: One is mental, and the other is physical. The same is true of erogenous zones, those areas of the human body that, when stimulated, lead to a sexual response. Although we usually think of erogenous zones in physical terms, in practice, the mind is a powerful erogenous zone that must be stimulated if the body is to experience its full pleasure potential. Only when mind and body are in perfect sexual synchronicity can a man reach the ultimate state of arousal. And guess what? You're the one holding the map to his erotic destination. So let's hit the road and get started on our journey.

Professional Skill versus Bedside Manner

David, a thirty-year-old single and seeking, understands the mind/body connection when it comes to stimulating a man's erogenous zones. He believes that more women should be conscious of it.

"I was with this woman for three years," David relates, "and she was incredible in bed. She had sexual techniques that would blow your mind and that most guys only fantasize about but never get to experience. It was like she wrote the book on the male body. She knew exactly where and when to suck, where and when to twist, where and when to push or pull. I've never, before or since, been with a woman who had such skill. She was a pro."

So why no wedding bells, you ask?

"She made me feel *good*," says David, "but I wanted to feel like a *god*. I know that sounds egocentric, but I think most men want to feel like sex gods. And if a woman gives him that feeling, well, it takes sex to a whole new level. This woman knew how to push the right buttons, but she never played to my ego or engaged my mind in sex. She was like a doctor who had great skill but terrible bedside manner." David laughs. "I always knew the operation would be successful, but I never really felt like she wanted me as a patient."

"I've had the other end of the spectrum as well," says David. "I've been with women who had a great bedside manner—they made me feel like a total stud—but who didn't really have the skill to match it. They said all the right things and would get me really worked up, but the sex itself didn't measure up. I guess that's just as unsatisfying."

If he had to choose between great bedside manner and "pro" sexual skill, which one would David pick?

"I honestly don't know," he admits. "I know lots of guys would take skill over bedside manner, but having had both, I'm not so sure. I love being turned on mentally as much as physically. That's why I'd tell women to focus on mental arousal along with the physical and to think of a man's mind as an erogenous zone, too."

Mind Games: Going from "Good" to "God"

Okay, so now that we know a man's mind is an erogenous zone, how do we put our knowledge into practice? How do we make our man feel not just good but godlike? Appealing to the male ego— the sexual ego in particular—is a good place to start. One of the easiest and most effective ways to inflate the male ego is to initiate sex more often. When a woman initiates sex, she makes her man feel desired, masculine, sexy, and irresistible.

A surefire way to stroke the male ego is to admire those areas of his body that aren't exactly sexual but that still pack mental and emotional punch.

Another way to stroke the male sexual ego is to focus your attention and admiration on those areas of your man's body that he may not consider to be sexual or erogenous but that still pack mental and emotional punch. Such areas include:

His face: Flatter your man by commenting on how handsome he is. This is an obvious yet often overlooked way to boost his ego and to make him feel sexually attractive and desirable.

His shoulders, arms, and hands: These zones are erogenous because they represent male physical strength. Why else would men instinctively flex their biceps when an attractive woman walks into the room? Complimenting your man on his strong shoulders, arms, and hands gives him confidence and makes him feel like the alpha male.

His back: Like the shoulders, arms, and hands, the back is associated with a man's sense of his own physical strength, masculinity, and self-confidence. A back massage feels wonderful to most men, but hearing a woman gush about his physique—how strong, smoothly muscled, and sexy his back is—feels just as good!

His chest: Second only to the penis, the chest is a symbol of virility and physical strength that is closely connected to a man's sense of power. Think of Tarzan pounding his iron chest in the jungle, communing with his inner primate. No, your guy might not swing from branch to branch beating his breast, but his chest is nonetheless the male equivalent of a peacock's feathers. Always sing the praises of your man's chest and let him know how much you admire it.

His hips and legs: A man's hips and legs may not be erogenous in the same way that his genitals are, but given their role in sexual activity—penetrating and thrusting—they are closely related to sexual power, stamina, and vitality. When you swoon at the sight of your partner's hips and legs, you make him feel desired and virile, like the sexual animal he is.

The Male Map

There are areas on a man's body that simply feel good when physically stimulated: A foot rub, for example, is pleasant and relaxing. Other areas feel more than good when stimulated, they feel sexual: A flick of the tongue on the inner thigh, for example, is electric and arousing. That's because, like a road map, a man's body has routes that lead to different destinations. Some are slow leisure trails that lead to pleasure zones, while others are sexual speedways that lead to erogenous zones. The question is which route to choose, the leisure trail or the sex speedway? Well, if you study the map, you'll find that both routes can take you where you want to go.

Pleasure Zones

As the saying goes, getting there is half the fun. Before you take the off-ramp to the sex speedway, why not spend some time traveling at a slower pace? It'll relax your partner and prepare his body for the bliss that is on the itinerary for later. Pleasure zones are those areas on a man's body that, while they may not elicit a strong erotic response, nonetheless feel luxurious and relaxing when stimulated.

The most common pleasure zones include:

His head, scalp, and face: Massaging and/or scratching your man's scalp stimulates blood circulation, which not only feels good but also helps to rid him of his worries and other distractions. A tender caress on his face while maintaining eye contact results in feelings of closeness and connection between you and your partner.

His shoulders, arms, and hands: Many men carry a significant amount of tension in their shoulders, often without even knowing it, making them appear hunched, tight, and stiff. A good shoulder rub can loosen these tense muscles and help lower the shoulders, which in turn relaxes the entire body. Massaging your man's hands, overworked and underpaid as they usually are, will make him feel soothed and indulged.

His back: Like the shoulders, the back is a storage facility for tension. Your man's back provides a large canvas upon which you can work to pleasurably relax him with a variety of massage strokes and caresses.

His legs and feet: You might rub your man's shoulders and back fairly regularly, but how often do you pay attention to his legs and feet? Yeah, that's what we thought. These oft-neglected body parts respond to massage with eager gratitude, so add them to the menu the next time you play masseuse.

His pleasure zones, at a glance:

- his head, scalp, and face
- his shoulders, arms, and hands
- his back
- his legs and feet

Sex or Sleep?

As you're winding your way through your man's pleasure zones, keep in mind that stimulating these areas of his body elicits a response that is very different from the one produced by stimulating his erogenous zones. Although many women find a back or foot rub to be highly erotic foreplay, many men find that stimulation of their pleasure zones leads to feelings of pure relaxation sans arousal.

The story of Jessy, a forty-two-year-old wife of ten years, shows how important it is to remember the pleasure-erogenous distinction when it comes to men. After a decade of marriage, her and her husband's sex life was something of a predictable routine: lights out, a squeeze under the covers, five minutes of the missionary, and then twenty minutes of the late show on television.

"I decided it was time to try something new in the bedroom," says Jessy. "Everybody's always talking about sensual massage, so I thought I'd try that. I probably spent half our retirement fund on scented massage oils, on so-called aphrodisiac love potions, aromatherapy, and essential oils that were supposed to turn him on. There was sweet almond, eucalyptus, grape seed oil, jojoba, you name it…if it sounded like a flower or a fruit, I rubbed it into his back."

And what happened?

"Nothing happened," Jessy reveals. "Ten minutes into a back rub, and his face would be buried in the pillow, his muffled snores sounding my defeat. There I was, trying to turn him on, rubbing our savings into his back, and he'd pass out without even a kiss. It was depressing. I took it personally. I felt like he was so bored with me, so turned off, that he'd rather sleep than have sex. That wasn't the guy I married."

But Jessy's fears were alleviated when she confronted her husband about his ill-timed sleep habits, asking why he had lost sexual interest in her.

"He just laughed," says Jessy. "He said that *he* was worried I was losing interest in *him*. He thought I was trying to put him to sleep with back rubs so that I didn't have to have sex with him. I told him the opposite was true: I was trying to turn him on with the back rubs. But he said that they were too relaxing to be arousing. So we made a plan. If I wanted to have sex, I'd rub his back in the nude, so that he could feel my nakedness on his back; that would be enough to keep him awake. It worked."

Jessy's experience is a caveat: Remember that pleasure zones relax, while erogenous zones arouse. As you're stimulating your man's soul-soothing pleasure zones, you can keep his attention by occasionally tossing out a sexy teaser. Jessy's solution to play the naked masseuse is a great idea. Some well-timed dirty talk will also do the trick. An unexpected and provocative suck on a finger or toe during a hand or foot massage will also work wonders; few men will fall asleep after such blatant allusions to fellatio!

Erogenous Zones

Once your man's pleasure zones have been explored, it's time to pick up sexual speed and steer to his erogenous zones. Erogenous zones are those areas of a man's body that, when stimulated, lead to a spike in erotic desire as well as a physical response in the form of sexual arousal.

Finding your man's erogenous zones is an erotic art, not a hard science. Every man is different: For example, one man may find his nipples to be a high-voltage erogenous zone, while others will have mediocre, negligible, or no sexual response to nipple stimulation. That being said, there are commonalities, and the areas suggested here are the ones you should definitely test to measure your man's unique sexual response.

The most common erogenous zones include:

His lips and mouth: Giving your man a kiss on his lips is the sweetest, simplest way to say "I love you and I desire you." Kissing is an intimate appetizer that lets him know sex that is on the menu. Stimulating the lips by kissing them or lightly tracing them with your fingertips elicits a sexual response, but don't forget the tongue's role in the action: It's an erogenous zone in its own right, and stimulating his tongue with your own increases eroticism, anticipation, and physical response. Stimulating the frenulum (the flap of tissue that connects the upper lip to the gums) may also turn on your man.

His ears: The ear area is packed with bundles of nerve endings that make it extremely sensitive. The earlobe, flap, and canal are highly responsive to erotic stimulation such as sucking, licking, nibbling, breath blowing, whispering, tongue penetrating, and so forth. The area behind his ear is also very sensitive, particularly as it leads down to the sides of his neck, another erogenous zone.

His neck: An exposed neck is as sexy as it is vulnerable. Who knows? Perhaps it's this element of instinctual, animalistic danger that makes neck stimulation so sexually arousing. The sides of your man's neck, the area of his Adam's apple, and the nape of his neck all respond strongly to erotic contact whether in the form of kissing, nibbling, or stroking.

His nipples: You know what it does for you, but what will nipple stimulation do for your man? As we've mentioned, nipple sensitivity in men runs the sexual gamut from hot to not. Give your man's nipples (and areolae) their due, and do your best to exploit this potentially powerful erogenous zone.

His sides: The stretch of skin alongside your man's body, from his armpits to his hips, is a large and ultrasensitive erogenous zone that responds well to stroking, licking, kissing, and caressing. The sides of a man's body aren't normally touched in a tender way (think of your poor guy sandwiched on the subway, his sides serving as bumpers against fellow passengers), and that may be one reason this area appreciates a softer touch.

His navel area: Your man's navel area, from his belly button to about where his pubic hair begins, is an erogenous zone not only because of its sensitivity but also because of its proximity to the genitals. This area is also home to the so-called treasure trail, the hairline that runs down a man's belly to his groin. The treasure trail is a sexy path that most men will appreciate your traveling.

His inner thighs: Your man's inner thighs don't usually receive a lot of stimulation and therefore respond strongly to erotic contact. Another reason for this strong reaction is the inner thigh's proximity to the groin. It's difficult to stimulate the inner thigh without grazing the genital region—whether with a brush of your hair or arm, or the feel of your breath—and the inadvertent contact causes spikes of intense sexual expectation.

His buttocks: Your man's buttocks provide a relatively large surface area of skin which responds eagerly to various types of erotic contact, from gentle caressing to strong squeezing, depending on your man's personal preferences. Spanking, for example, is an activity that increases blood flow to the buttocks and that many men enjoy for both the mental aspect as well as the physical burn. Like other parts of the body (the sides and inner thighs, in particular), the buttocks don't normally receive a lot of erotic attention—after all, they spend most of their time stuck in a chair—and, again, because of this neglect they appreciate attention. For the man who enjoys anal play, stimulating the buttocks makes him crave and anticipate anal contact.

His anal area: Your man's anal area is loaded with nerve endings and is exceptionally responsive to physical stimulation. That being said, there are many cultural forces at work that may prevent a heterosexual man from exploring this erogenous zone. The topic of anal play, including proper stimulation of the prostate gland (below), is covered in later chapters (particularly chapters 4, 6, 8, 9, and 10).

The prostate gland: The prostate gland, the male equivalent of the female G-spot, is located a few inches inside the rectum, on the anterior or front-facing wall. Proper stimulation of the prostate gland results in feelings of intense sexual pleasure.

His genitals and groin area: Your man's genitals—his penis and testicles—are the most sensitive and powerful erogenous zones on his body, the ones directly involved in orgasm and ejaculation. Your man's genitals, as well as his entire groin area, boast a number of distinct and powerful hot spots, from his glans penis and frenulum to his scrotal sac and perineum. Stimulation of these erog-

 His erogenous zones, at a glance:

- his lips and mouth
- his ears
- his neck
- his nipples
- his sides
- his navel area
- his inner thighs
- his buttocks
- his anal area and prostate gland
- his genitals and groin area

enous zones provides unparalleled sexual sensation and pleasure. The specific location of these genital/groin erogenous zones, as well as ways to stimulate them, will be discussed in later chapters (particularly chapters 6, 8, 9, and 10).

The Unmarked Roads

The distinction between a pleasure zone and an erogenous zone is a highly subjective one. As we've said, finding your man's erogenous zones is an erotic art, not a hard science, and there will be areas on the male map where the roads between general physical pleasure and actual sexual arousal are unmarked. The distinction between pleasure zones and erogenous zones is made even more difficult by the fact that, for a woman, almost *any* area of the body can be erogenous. After all, we are the more sensitive sex!

For example, a kiss or similar stimulation to a closed eyelid, palm, inside crook of the elbow, back of the knee, or shoulder may elicit sexual feelings in women, while resulting in nonsexual yet pleasurable feelings in men. Stimulation of these areas may also result in the best of both worlds, where your man experiences an overlap of sexual and nonsexual feelings.

All Roads Lead to Rome

In the end, it's up to you to read the male map and to see where each road—mental and physical, marked and unmarked—may lead.

Just as all roads led to Rome, there are many different routes to reach the state of arousal and to prepare your man's mind and body to receive both a full-body kiss and fellatio. And when you take the time and effort to study the map and find the most scenic routes, your man will enjoy the journey as much as the destination.

3 : Setting the Mood

The art of oral sex isn't just about learning a new mouth move or tongue twist. It's also about seduction, about bringing your man to a pure, heightened state of arousal where he can fully experience the erotic power of your mouth as a sexual organ. Learning the art of dirty talk and studying his body's erogenous zones enable you to mentally and physically arouse your man, but before you can put your knowledge into practice and perform a full-body kiss and fellatio, you must set the mood for these erotic events.

The mood or sensual aura that surrounds the performance of oral pleasure can greatly affect how much or how little sexual enjoyment your man receives from the experience. If you're dressed in one of his ratty oversized sweatshirts, the dog is scratching to get into the bedroom, and the television is blaring some documentary on the fecal content of fast food, he may not be entirely focused on what's happening sexually. Therefore it's vital to set a mood that will complement and enhance the oral-sex experience rather than one that will distract from or dilute it.

Sex and the Senses

During an intimate encounter, a woman's body engages all five of a man's senses—sight, sound, smell, touch, and taste—to varying degrees. The way a woman prepares her body therefore creates a sensual aura that both sets the mood for sex and gets her man in the mood for sex. Because your body has the potential to be a sensorial delight to your man, always keep the following basic points in mind:

During sex, a woman's body engages all of a man's senses, including sight, sound, smell, touch, and taste. To exploit this feast of the senses, always prepare your body for sex.

TOUCH The feel of a woman's soft skin moving and pressing against their body is a powerful turn-on for men. To exploit this fact, always make sure to shave or wax so that your skin is smooth and feminine. Equally important is a good moisturizer to ensure that your soft, supple body feels exquisite to him. (Be sure to pay particular attention to those dry patches on the elbows, knees, and heels). Warming lotions add sizzle and can really heat things up—he'll think he's on fire! And keep your fingernails long enough to deliver a sexy cat scratch to his back at just the right moment.

SIGHT Men are very visual and easily aroused by erotic imagery. That fact begs the question: What is your man usually looking at during sex? That's right. Your body. It's eye candy. To make it as sweet as possible, hit the lingerie shop and deck yourself out in the designs that will both flatter your figure and excite your man. The sexy smoothness of stockings, even without an attendant garter belt, will appeal to both his touch and sight. The appearance of your pubic hair is also important. Does your man prefer it au naturale, groomed, or smooth? The way you move your body can also play a part in visual arousal. A sultry walk across the bedroom or a sexy crawl over the bed is a visual invitation he'll eagerly accept.

TASTE Since your body is eye candy, it should taste delicious. Always make sure to use mouthwash before engaging in any sexual activity with your man and, to add an extra zing to kisses, wear a flavored lip balm. Apply some of the flavored lip balm to your nipples to make them sugary sweet, too. The range of edible/flavored massage lotions and oils as well as flavored lubricants now available is wide enough to suit any taste. Chocolate body paint, flavored body powders/dust, and whipped cream are other sexy snacks you can serve on bare skin.

SOUND As discussed in chapter 1, The Art of Dirty Talk, certain sounds can increase the level of a man's sexual desire. Remember the lessons of that chapter and use your word choice and tone as well as your moans, sighs, and the rhythm of your breathing to arouse your man and set an erotic mood for sex.

SMELL Perfume is an obvious choice when it comes to scenting your body, but there are other options, too. For example, you can use a fragrant body lotion when you moisturize. This allows you to scent every inch of your skin and to experiment with different fragrances to see which one your man likes best. A scented shampoo is also a must, since many men love the smell of a woman's hair, particularly when she's fresh from the shower.

Location, Location, Location

What image comes to mind when you think of setting the mood for sex? A candle-lit bedroom? Red rose petals sprinkled on the sheets and the scent of aromatherapy in the air? *Zzzzzz*...Recognize that sound? It's the sound of your man sleeping. Sure, the scent of lavender linen spray may turn you on, but it may not have the same warming effect on your man's libido. Lucky for him, then, that the arts of full-body kissing and fellatio aren't limited to the bedroom—and don't require rose petals.

That being said, the bedroom does have its advantages. That bed sure is soft, isn't it? And it's soooo nice to just roll over and fall asleep when the deed is done. Even more important for those with kids or houseguests, the door has a lock. But other areas have advantages, too. The sheer sexual novelty of receiving oral sex beyond the borders of his bedroom can add real excitement to your man's experience.

The novelty of receiving oral sex beyond his bedroom walls can add excitement to your man's experience.

The bathroom, for example, offers the perfect location for steamy oral sex. Pour some bubble bath into the tub, slip into the water, and lie against your man's body, covering your breasts with the bubbles until they all pop and he has a full view. You can stay in the water while he sits on the side of the bathtub so that you can perform oral sex like a mischievous mermaid. Or you can drain the tub and have him lie naked on the bottom while your wet, naked body works on him from above.

Another aquatic option is to share a shower and satisfy him while he stands and you kneel in front of him. As you'll read in the chapters on full-body kissing and fellatio, oral sex can be performed while your partner is in a number of positions.

Just remember that a change of location doesn't have to be anything dramatic. After all, it's the elements of variety and unfamiliarity that make the experience so thrilling, not the different pictures that line the walls. Believe it or not, even the hallway floor can be a fun, sexy place to perform a full-body kiss and fellatio: The feel of carpet under your naked bodies, the strangeness of being so low, the closeness of the walls, and the sense of exhibitionism all come together to make a hallway-floor sex session an exciting alternative to that comfy king-size bed of yours.

Take a stroll through your house and think about which areas you haven't christened yet. The staircase? Your man can recline on the steps while you work on him from below, slowly snaking your way up between his legs. The garage? The hood or backseat of the car gives you plenty of room for a sexy automotive adventure. The camper parked in the driveway? You don't have to head to the hills to have a romp. The backyard? Privacy and weather permitting, having sex under the stars is absolute heaven.

While you as a woman may prefer to receive something as sensual as a full-body kiss and oral sex in the familiar comfort and relaxing serenity of your boudoir, the same may not always hold true for your man. While a bedroom body-kiss and oral-sex session—complete with lavender linen spray on the sheets—can be a luxuriously tranquil experience for him, don't be afraid to indulge his sense of erotic adventure now and then. The sky's the limit when it comes to lusty locations, so don't always lock your-selves behind bedroom doors.

Passion Props

Passion props are anything you use to set the stage for an unforget-table oral-sex experience. (This doesn't include the use of sex toys, which is the subject of chapter 9.) Of course, the props you use depend on the location you've chosen.

If you're in the living room, you can use your man's favorite recliner. He can sit back in comfort while you kneel in front of the chair. If you're in the kitchen, you can use the table. He can lie on top while you feast on him. Oh come on, why not? Spread out the tablecloth and serve him something different. Almost *anything* out of the ordinary heightens arousal and adds a novel sense of exhil-aration to the encounter, so use your imagination and work with what you have.

Mirrors are easy and effective props that can bring an exciting visual dimension to fellatio. The sight of being sucked and licked is an incredibly potent one: Your man won't be able to tear his eyes away from the magic show in the mirror.

To make the show even better, turn the lights up. While most women find low lighting to be more sensual, many men love having sex with the lights on. If you're normally a lights-out kind of girl, surprise your guy and leave the switch on while you perform oral sex; it's the perfect opportunity, especially since you don't have to be completely undressed for the performance.

Adult movies may also appeal to your man's visual nature, and the wide variety of films currently available allows you to set whatever kind of mood you wish for oral sex. Hard-core, male-focused movies will set a raunchy mood that your partner may enjoy, particularly if you and he normally choose more couple-friendly pornography. Soft-core porn, including those movies made for the couples' market and instructional sex videos on erotic massage or sexual positions, will create a softer, more erotic mood.

As we learned in chapter 1, the sounds of sex can also excite a man and create an electrifying aura. If you're opposed to (or just bored with) visual pornography, there are erotic CDs that offer a fun, fresh alternative to visual porn. The explicit stories and sounds—all those moans, groans, grunts, and heavy sighs—set a sexually charged background not only for a full-body kiss and fellatio but also for lovemaking. Audio erotica is second to none when it comes to firing up the libido and engaging the imagination. It is available online to order or download and is also sold in some sex shops.

Furniture, mirrors, bright lighting, and various forms of porn are all potential passion props.

Online pornography can also be used as a passion prop while you are orally pleasuring your partner. You can have your man surf the Internet and take a few "free tours" of sex sites, or you can go all the way and let him engage in anonymous cybersex, with or without a webcam. The feel of your mouth on his body and genitals while he participates in such alluring activities will bring a taboo thrill to his oral-sex experience.

Like audio erotica, cybersex brings a new dimension to the porn experience by allowing you and/or your partner to participate in the action. This activity, however, is not for everyone, and you should discuss it with your man before introducing cybersex into your love life. If it's territory you're unsure about entering, it's best to stay away. There are more than enough ways to spice up a sex life without wading into waters you're not completely confident about.

"Rock Star" Sex

Music is another excellent passion prop. It has an uncanny ability to influence and enhance our emotions, and, with a little thought, you can choose the music that will create exactly the mood you want.

Luke, twenty-eight, explains why his fiancée, Sara, formerly a low-decibel lover, is now the master of mood music: "We'd always had sex in silence," says Luke, "no music, no television, nothing. I guess we thought it would be too distracting. But that changed when we moved into our new house. We had a big garage party for everybody who had helped move us in. The music was loud, and some guys were fooling around with an old electric guitar they'd come across. When the party ended, Sara and I were still wired. We started fooling around right there in the garage, with the music still blaring. It was really different. I kept expecting her to turn the music off and lead me into the bedroom, but she didn't."

"I was sitting on a speaker when Sara suddenly knelt in front of me and unzipped my jeans," continues Luke. "She started sucking me right there, like she couldn't help herself. I felt like a rock star. The music was pounding in my ears, and I was being sucked off. It was nasty. I can honestly say that's the first time I've had sex like that, where a fantasy completely took hold of me and I lived it out. I often have fantasies go through my head when we're having sex, but that's the first time it played out so perfectly. I was the rock star and she was the groupie. It was great."

Okay, so Sara hit the mark that time, but is her aim still as good?

"Sara's the reigning queen of sex tunes," Luke boasts. "After she saw how much I enjoyed playing the rock star, she started to experiment with all kinds of music in our sex life. Sometimes it's slow and sweet, sometimes fast and nasty. One of my favorites is this drumming music she has, some exotic-sounding tribal CD she found at a yard sale. The rhythmic beat of the drums puts us into this dazed, almost out-of-body state where we just move and thrust to the music. It's an incredible experience."

Music is therefore an easy and exciting way to set the mood for sex; however, as Sara knows, it's important to change the station now and then so you don't get stuck in the same groove. Sample different types of tunes to see which ones will create the background sounds you're looking for.

It's Only Make-Believe

Luke's rock-star role play shines the spotlight on a fantastic way to set the mood for oral sex and seduction: exploiting male sexual fantasies. Appealing to your man's wet dreams is a foolproof way to get him in the mood for a "make-believe" blow job. Scan the five role-play possibilities below to see if their plots might intrigue him. The sequels are for you to write!

 Immersing your man in his favorite sexual fantasy can set a fiery mood for fellatio.

THE RED-LIGHT DISTRICT Paying for sex is a popular male fantasy. To make this dream come true, put a red lightbulb into a night-light and plug it into your bedroom wall or drape a red fabric over a lamp shade. This turns your boudoir into an exotic, enticing red-light district. Smooth a cool satin sheet onto the mattress and step into a call-girl corset, perhaps accented with a choker, long satin gloves, a garter belt with stockings, and stiletto heels. Playing a XXX film in the background completes the transformation to give your man the biggest bang for his buck. And don't break character. Ask him what he wants, tell him what it costs, and then give it to him. Have your man pay you with real money, too. The physical act of handing over the cash will give this sexy scene an authentic aura.

UP AGAINST A WALL Anonymity is also a favorite element of many male fantasies. Turn down the lights, push your man against a wall, and frantically strip him. Tell him to imagine he's receiving a quickie blow job in an alley from a stranger he just met at the bar. It's pitch-black out, and he can't even remember what the woman looks like. In addition to the anonymity, the standing-up-against-a-wall position brings a deliciously nasty quality to this quickie.

LAUNDRY-ROOM LOVERS This fantasy boasts four powerfully erotic elements: the novelty of sex in an unfamiliar place, the thrill of sex with a stranger, the excitement of exhibitionism, and the danger of getting caught. Lead your man into your laundry room and take off his clothes. Next, have him sit with spread legs on the washer—the spin cycle is best—so that the vibrations can bring an extra buzz to his blow job. Tell him to pretend he's at an empty, all-night laundromat receiving oral sex from the only other patron in the store, while passersby peek through the windows. The problem is that his wife/girlfriend could walk through the door at any moment...

BLOW JOBS FOR BEGINNERS The idea of receiving oral sex from an inexperienced woman is an exciting prospect for many men. They love the thought of their manhood being the first she'll have in her mouth. How will she suck? How will she react when he ejaculates? Will she swallow it? Of course, men love a skillful blow job, but there's also something enticing about inexperience. In this role play, you assume the character of an eager but inexperienced woman who wants to learn how to perform fellatio. Your man plays the part of the stud who teaches her, step by step and suck by suck, how to satisfy a man. Pretend that you've never done it before, and tell your man to put his hands on your head while you practice. Encourage him to talk you through the tutorial by telling you when to lick, nibble, twist, stroke, and suck. And be sure to follow his directions with all the enthusiasm of a naughty novice.

THE POWER STRUGGLE If good-girl innocence fueled the last fantasy, bad-girl sinfulness drives this one. Many men are turned on by the idea of being helplessly used and pleasured—sometimes against their will—by a woman. This role play dips into the sexual practice of bondage to satisfy this craving. To bring the fantasy to life, choose a way to restrain your man. You can tie him to a chair, handcuff him to the headboard, or simply wrap a scarf or a necktie around his wrists and/or ankles; there's no need to purchase BDSM (Bondage, Domination and Submission, Sadism, and Masochism) bondage gear! When he's in place, you can begin to assault his body and genitals with pleasure, doing whatever you wish to him while he's in this helpless state. Using sex toys on your man during this fantasy would add a thrilling dimension, so keep this role play in mind after you've read the chapter on sex toys (chapter 9).

Incidentally, you and your partner may want to agree on a "safe" word before you begin this fantasy. This should be a word you don't normally say during sex, like *antelope* or *linoleum*. If your man wants to be untied at any time during the fantasy, he can say the word, and you'll know the game's over.

Smile and the World Smiles with You

While this chapter offers some great ways to set the mood for a full-body kiss and fellatio, it is ultimately *your* mood that will determine the sensual aura that accompanies the experience. Your attitude is paramount. It's also infectious. If you're not enthusiastic about what you're doing, your man will notice, and his pleasure will plummet. On the other hand, if you approach oral sex and seduction with genuine affection and eager sexual joy, you'll maximize your partner's enjoyment. A smile sets the sexiest mood of all, so flash your ivories and let him know how good his pleasure makes you feel.

4 The Art of Full-Body Kissing

When you think about it, a kiss is an amazing thing. As a form of human interaction, it has incredible dimension in terms of use, meaning, expression, emotion, and symbolism. Kisses have been used to heal, to marry, and to betray. They seal deals and, if the kisses are forbidden, break unions. Both politicians and parents kiss babies, but even an infant can recognize the difference between the coolness of a "vote-for-me" kiss and the warmth of a "you-are-my-child" kiss.

We kiss at the arrival gate in happy greeting, and we kiss at the departure gate in sad good-bye. We kiss hands and rings to show respect and deference. We kiss the ground after a rough flight to show relief. We kiss ass to get ahead. We kiss our lovers, children, parents, friends, associates, enemies, and even our pets. We blow kisses through the air, and we send XOs in the mail or via text message. All this kissing, and yet we never forget our first one. Indeed, the kiss is the little black dress of human interaction; it has a thousand uses.

A kiss's greatest purpose is the physical, emotional, and sexual bond it creates between lovers. Lovers have their own inventory of kisses, from the morning good-bye peck on the cheek to the midnight kiss on the mouth. When a woman kisses her man lightly on the end of his nose, she expresses playful affection for him. When she kisses him deeply on the lips, she expresses passionate lust for him. The meanings of a lover's kiss are therefore many and varied: I love you, I missed you, I need you, I forgive you, I want you.

 A full-body kiss is the ultimate lover's kiss, at once expressing love, adoration, and desire.

A full-body kiss is the ultimate lover's kiss. By rapturously encompassing every inch of a lover's body, it allows the giver to express her profound love, erotic adoration, and sexual desire for her partner while at the same time immersing the receiver in a state of pure ecstasy. A full-body kiss is therefore a blissful form of foreplay to both lovemaking and fellatio; but it serves a higher purpose, too, by creating and maintaining a special bond between lovers that no other kiss can match in either emotional intensity or physical intimacy.

The Full-Body Bond

The rocky romance of Maggie and Chris, together for five years but just recently wed, illustrates the bonding potential of the full-body kiss. Chris, a self-admitted workaholic, traveled extensively out of town on business, a trend that only worsened when the couple exchanged their vows. As if Chris's deliberate absenteeism weren't enough to put a strain on the relationship, Maggie's secret coping strategy for those lonely nights—sharing her bed with a standing selection of willing ex-boyfriends—added extra poison to an already toxic mix.

"Chris was gone for days at a time," says Maggie, "sometimes for a week or more, depending on where he was going and what project he was working on. I thought that once we got married he'd slow down and be home more, but the opposite happened. I took it personally. The more nights he spent away, the more I felt like he wasn't attracted to me, like he didn't even care if we had sex or not. So I turned to guys that I knew wanted to sleep with me."

But was Maggie's assessment true? Was Chris uninterested in sex with his wife?

"Our sex life was okay," says Chris. "Maggie's a beautiful woman, and I knew that she'd had a lot of sexual partners before we got together. If I'm totally honest, that was always in the back of my mind, even in the beginning. A guy wants to feel like he's the best lay his girl's ever had, but I never felt that way. I felt like I was nothing special. That's hard on a guy's ego and even worse on the libido. I wondered how I compared to the others, and I always assumed I fell short. My reaction was to physically withdraw."

Meanwhile, Maggie had initiated contact with yet another ex-boyfriend. The contact soon spread from cyberspace to the local coffeehouse and then, inevitably, to the bedroom. This ex-boyfriend, however, didn't prove to be as discreet as his predecessors, and a wayward e-mail found its way into Chris and Maggie's shared account.

"I felt my stomach sink, and I could feel the rage rising in my throat as I read the e-mail," says Chris. "It was beyond horrible. This guy was saying how good it was, how he couldn't wait to see her again, and asking when I'd be out of town next. There was no mistaking what was going on. I felt sick, disgusted, betrayed. I filed for divorce."

"We went through all the motions of a divorce," says Maggie. "We had lawyers, court dates, papers. It was the most depressing time of my life. And it was only then, at the end of our relationship, that I realized how much Chris meant to me. I guess that's the way it usually happens. I realized that I'd always taken him for granted."

"I'd taken Maggie for granted, too," Chris admits. "Why else would I leave her alone so much? When I look back, I think that I was trying to punish her for her past by being away. I knew she was highly sexed, so withholding sex was a power thing. I used it to get back at her for making me feel second rate in the bedroom. No, she didn't make me feel that way on purpose. It was the combination of her past and my insecurities that led to those feelings."

Unexpectedly, it was Maggie's lawyer who, at the eleventh hour, stepped in to stave off divorce.

"She knew that I didn't want the divorce, and she suggested that we go to counseling," explains Maggie. "I didn't expect Chris to agree, but he did."

"I didn't think I'd ever forgive Maggie," says Chris, "and I'm still working on that. It sounds crazy, but despite her affairs, we're more a real couple now than we were before. Therapy might not work for everyone, but it did help us understand one another and recommit to our marriage."

Okay, so counseling helped this couple understand and commit to each other. But what about their sex life? If Chris and Maggie's bedroom thermostat was set on cool *before* the string of infidelities, didn't the temperature drop even more in their aftermath?

"Initially, yes," admits Chris. "I couldn't even think about having sex with her. All I could do was picture her rolling around naked with some guy. Even worse, I had a hard time convincing myself that she was really attracted to me."

But did things improve?

"Things got better very slowly," Chris continues. "Time took care of the first problem—the pictures in my head. My feelings of sexual inadequacy took longer to fix. I felt like she was thinking about other men. That made it difficult to get close."

"I tried to initiate sex a thousand times, but he'd always pull back," says Maggie. "I had to find a way to show him how special he was, how much I desired him. He had to believe that I found his body irresistible, head to toe."

Trying to regain a lover's trust and affection after infidelity is no small task, and, as Maggie discovered, reestablishing their intimate bond would take more than time. It would take real heartfelt effort on her part.

"We were lying in bed, holding hands, when I kissed him on the back of his hand. He didn't pull away, so I continued to kiss his fingers, then along his arm, down his chest, over his stomach, and down his legs. I didn't even try to go for his genitals. I kept it sweet and undemanding. I kissed every inch of his body, treating each kiss like an apology and a promise. As each minute passed, I was more surprised that he wasn't pushing me away."

"It was the first time I'd felt so special," says Chris. "She wasn't trying to get me hard or get herself off, she was just covering my body in wonderful feelings. She was just pampering me, and I felt... this sounds ridiculous... but I felt like she was *worshipping* my body. After our history, I needed to feel that way. For me, it was the only way I could regain sexual confidence and know that she wanted me."

"That whole-body kiss was really a bonding exercise for us," Maggie explains. "It brought us back together physically and sexually as well as emotionally. Those things are all wound up together in an intimate relationship, and a whole-body kiss is all of those things. It's a physical and sexual act, but it's very emotional, too. Our therapist had suggested we try sensual massage for the same reason, but for us the whole-body kiss was even more intimate and erotic."

"It was her mouth that made it so intimate," says Chris. "Sensual massage is great, too, but the body kiss just seemed more personal. It brought our bodies closer together than massage did, and the feel of her lips on my skin broke through all our barriers. To us, whole-body kissing is even more bonding than intercourse, and it's made our relationship tighter than ever."

Full-Body Fun

A full-body kiss does more than offer a couple a way to physically, sexually, and emotionally bond. It also offers them a fun, sexy way to add erotic anticipation to their sex life. Whatever its positive side effects on the relationship as a whole may be, the full-body kiss is first and foremost a passion-filled way to play and to prep your man for fellatio.

"I've had my share of sex," laughs Leah, twenty-nine. "I'm the quintessential swinging single. I love sex, but I'd be lying if I said it didn't get predictable. For the most part, everybody does the same things. I'd look at a guy and think, 'Wow, he looks like he'd be a stallion,' but then it'd be the same bump and grind. And even worse, I know that I pull the same moves all the time. I'd be horrified to find out that a guy found me boring in bed. That'd be the ultimate insult."

Sexual boredom—the ultimate lover's insult—needn't be inevitable, even for the most active of the sexually active. But adding variety to one's sexual repertoire doesn't have to include studying the kama sutra, twisting oneself into a series of new sexual positions, investing in a warehouse of sex toys, or diving into a world of whips and chains. True sexual skill is measured by the level of arousal you can elicit from your partner, and a full-body kiss is a potent way to increase any man's libido.

> True sexual skill is measured by how well you can arouse your man, and a full-body kiss is a potent way to fire up his libido.

"The idea of body kissing seemed too simple to be sexy," Leah admits, "but I was amazed by how well it worked on my last boyfriend. I'd never seen a man so completely captivated by what I was doing. I spent the better part of an hour seducing him with the body kiss, and when I finally got to the blow job, he blew like a humpback whale. I've never seen a guy so ready. The body kiss made him drunk with anticipation for what was coming."

As foreplay to fellatio, the full-body kiss is second to none. The buildup to sex—all that teasing and delayed gratification—is often as pleasurable as the final sexual release, so be sure to extend your man's erotic expectation as long as possible before diving "down there." Not only will you dodge sexual boredom, you'll also make his cup of arousal runneth over.

The Mouth as a Sexual Organ

Now that we appreciate the power of the full-body kiss, we can turn our attention to its performance. To perfect the art of full-body kissing, a woman must begin to think of her mouth as more than just a set of lips. She must think of her mouth as a sex organ, as an instrument capable of expressing her erotic emotions while at the same time providing physical pleasure to her partner.

Your mouth has the potential to be the sexiest part of your body. It also has the ability to elicit the strongest sexual response from your man's body. Whether it's through the words you speak to him (recall those dirty-language lessons in chapter 1), the kisses you cover his body with, or the way your lips stroke his shaft, you must think of your mouth as a sex organ and learn to play it like a master.

Lip Lingerie

Just as you emphasize the seductive beauty of your body by adorning it in lingerie, so, too, can you exploit your mouth's passion potential by dressing it up. The same way that your moisturized arms and stockinged legs feel smoothly sexy wrapped around your lover's body, your well-moisturized lips will feel smooth and sexy against his skin. Effective moisturizing is therefore the first step to preening your puckers for a full-body kiss. After all, what man wants to be caressed by sandpaper?

To keep your lips soft and supple, drink plenty of water, avoid licking your lips excessively, use a gentle facial cleanser, and follow up with a good moisturizer. There are plenty of moisturizers designed specifically for the lips, so add one to the bottles of creams, serums, and lotions that line your bathroom cabinet. Choose a non-drying lipstick during the day, and, if your lipstick doesn't contain one, slap on a good moisturizing balm with an SPF of 15 or 30.

If your lips are in need of emergency exfoliation, apply some lip cream to a toothbrush and scrub lightly. There is a plethora of products available for this purpose, but before you part with big bucks for a small tube of brand-name lip buffer, consider this: My grandmother used to exfoliate with good ol' petroleum jelly and a washcloth. Even at eighty, she had the lips of a schoolgirl.

While you probably have a small army of lipsticks at your command, you may not have the same reserve when it comes to lip balm, but an assortment of differently flavored lip balms is as essential to your mouth as a selection of lingerie is to your body. Make sure the balm is colorless so that it doesn't leave pink streaks on your partner's skin, and try to select nonwaxy types to facilitate smoother travels along his body. Mix up the balm you wear to bed—strawberry flavored one night, spearmint the next—to keep your kisses fresh, tasty, and exciting.

To maximize the power of your pout, you can also try using a nonsurgical lip plumper. As with any other beauty product, the vast selection will have you standing in the cosmetics aisle for most of the afternoon, reading labels and trying to decipher the ingredients. Some lip plumpers claim to increase collagen production; others just smooth the lips. Some are for daytime use under makeup; others are nighttime treatments. Since what works for your sister may not work for you, there's no way to say which product is best, so buyer beware. If you're planning to wear the product to bed, however, ask the beauty consultant for a tester so you can see how gooey the goods are. A sticky kiss isn't sexy.

Mouth Maintenance

Now do a teeth check. When was the last time you had your teeth cleaned and polished? Could whitening, even with one of those home kits, make your smile brighter? Do you use mouthwash before bed, or do you cut corners by expecting your toothpaste to pick up the slack? Is your pack of dental floss so old that it belongs in the National Museum of Dentistry? (Yes, there is one. I checked.) Does your toothbrush have a proper tongue cleaner or scraper to rid itself of bacteria while reducing bad breath?

It might not sound sexy, but good oral hygiene plays a big role in attraction. We'll prove it. Picture cozying up to the man of your dreams. Now picture him trying to kiss you with puffy red gums, a spinach-toothed yellow smile, and halitosis that could drop-kick a horse. Are you cringing? Of course you are. And men are just as turned off by women whose smiles don't shine.

Remember that your mouth holds as much sex appeal as any other body part, so before you practice the art of oral pleasure, practice some mouth maintenance. It'll give you oral confidence, and it'll make your kisser even more kissable. After all, a healthy smile is a sexy smile.

The Three Ss: Sweet, Sinful, and Sultry

Now that your lips are dressed to kill and your mouth is squeaky clean, you're ready to embark on the full-body kiss. The first thing you'll have to consider is what style of body kiss you want to perform. While each style will arouse your man, each also creates a unique erotic aura that will have a distinctly different effect on his libido. Choosing the right style of body kiss and maintaining that style for the entire performance is essential if you wish to perfect the art of full-body kissing.

There are three styles from which to choose:

Sweet: The sweet style of body kissing is gentle and romantic. It can soothe your man's troubled mind, de-stress his body, help heal emotional wounds, and strengthen the bond between you. This heavenly kiss will make him think you're an angel.

Sinful: This naughty style of full-body kissing is perfect for a night of nasty, dirty oral sex. It is best performed when you're feeling sexually aggressive or want to show your man what a she-devil you can be. This bad-girl body kiss is pure raunch.

Sultry: Passionate, slow-burning, and very seductive, the sultry style of body kissing is ideal for those evenings you want to unleash your inner sexual temptress to play the role of the classic sexual minx.

Please Make Your Selection Now

Once you're familiar with the styles of full-body kisses available, how do you choose the one that's right for you and your partner? Your choice depends on many things, some of which include your and your man's sexual cravings, mood, level and quality of desire, life and relationship circumstances, erotic aura, sexual pattern or routine, and how much time you have to devote to the kiss.

For example, if your partner has recently suffered a loss in his life, you may want to nurse him with a sweet smothering of kisses. Sexual contact and feelings can be erotically nurturing if shared with someone you truly love. A sweet style is also perfect for make-up sex; the combination of strong emotions and tender caresses is a powerful formula for forgiveness.

If you and your man have just returned from a heart-pounding horror flick, you may wish to monopolize the adrenalin pumping through your veins and attack his flesh with the blazing, blood-thirsty intensity of a sinful full-body kiss. Or, if you're celebrating your anniversary and want to prove that you're the same femme fatale he married, you may choose to flaunt your sexual skill by subjecting him to the sheet-clutching agony and ecstasy of an all-night, sultry full-body kiss.

Variety is also something to consider. Once you've introduced the full-body kiss into your love life, you should keep a mental note of what style or styles you've recently used. Repeatedly falling back on the same style will dull its impact and make the experience predictable for your partner. Shake up the styles you use to keep your partner guessing. It'll ensure that the full-body kiss remains a potent form of foreplay to oral sex.

Another important factor to remember when making your style selection is the mood you've set from the previous chapter. Are you decked out in dominatrix attire, or are you under wraps in an innocent white cotton nightgown? Is there loud rock music pounding in the background, or have you created a more classical aura? Are you luxuriously stretched out on your king-size bed, or are you crowded into the backseat of your car? Is pornography adding viewing pleasure to the experience, and, if so, is it hard-core or erotic? These are the types of questions you should ask yourself before you choose a style of full-body kiss.

 The style of body kiss you choose should always suit the mood you've set.

Style and mood should always be complementary: A naughty red negligee goes well with a sinful style; romantic music suits a sweet style; a large Jacuzzi tub is a steamy spot to host a sultry style. A preplanned and well-orchestrated body kiss results in a five-star performance that no man will want to miss, so think ahead to make sure you receive the accolades you deserve.

My husband has asked me to start role-playing his sexual fantasies. Some of them involve women he picks up for one-night stands. Do you think these fantasies are cheating?

♀ *Debra:* In my opinion, sharing sexual fantasies isn't infidelity. I think this type of sharing can be healthy, fun, and bring variety into your sex life. Don't read too much into your husband's fantasies, and try not to be ultrasensitive to them. The kind of fantasy you've described sounds fairly tame. Unless his fantasies start to include creepier elements (such as underage partners, animals, violence), I think you're okay.

♂ *Don:* Your husband is completely normal. You should be thrilled that he's talking to you about his fantasies, and join in the fun. As long as his one-night stands remain imaginary, there's nothing wrong with where his mind is going. Remember that it's the idea of an anonymous one-night stand that's turning him on, not another real woman.

The Fantasy Factor

Male sexual fantasy is another factor that will influence the kissing style you choose. In the last chapter, you learned to exploit your man's secret sexual desires and erotic imagination by immersing him in a sexual fantasy. Let's quickly revisit these role plays to decide which kissing styles suit which sexy scenes.

Depending on the spin you put on the "facts" of the fantasy, the Laundry-Room Lovers story can use any of the three styles. Are the characters complete strangers and acting in lusty haste? How sinful. Have they been admiring each other for weeks, longing to be close and finally daring to touch? Oh, how sweet. Has the woman been eyeing the man all night, doing her best to tempt him while his girlfriend is gone? That's she-devil sultry.

The Red-Light District's raunchy, paying-for-it, XXX atmosphere makes this fantasy the perfect pick for a sinful style of full-body kissing; however, this scene can also support a sultry style if you choose to play the part of a highly-paid, highly-qualified escort as opposed to a curbside call girl. The Power Struggle fantasy has similar versatility and can also support either the sinful or sultry styles, again depending on the role you want to play. Do you want to dominate and make it hurt a little, or do you just want to show off your skills?

The Up Against a Wall and Blow Jobs for Beginners fantasies support only one style. The anonymity and "quickie" quality of Up Against a Wall is ideally suited to the sinful style, while the innocence and inexperience of Blow Jobs for Beginners is the perfect platform for the sweet style.

The Case for Consistency

After you've chosen the style of full-body kiss you wish to deliver, the next step is to recognize the importance of consistency of style.

Think of a singer performing a song or a dancer performing a dance. A sultry jazz singer seduces her listener with a slow, sexy style; how unpleasant would it be if, midsong, she suddenly started screeching out a heavy-metal tune? A woman in the dramatic throes of dancing the tango has her partner's heart pounding with raw sexual energy; wouldn't it derail his libido if she suddenly started square-dancing? Just as consistency of style is necessary in music and dance, so, too, is it essential when practicing the art of full-body kissing.

A singer selects the song she wants to sing and then carries the tune until the song ends. A dancer chooses the dance she wants to perform and then proceeds to do so until the music stops. Likewise, a lover chooses the style of full-body kiss she wants to engage in and then maintains that kiss's particular erotic aura until her mouth has moved over every part of her lover's body.

Such kissing consistency ensures that your man's arousal increases at a steady, regular rate that will prepare his body for fellatio. Consistency of style also helps you concentrate on what you're doing, so that you don't hit a bad note or miss a beat during your performance. It helps you focus on each specific part of the body kiss while seamlessly integrating it into the whole experience, thereby carrying out the kiss with skill, fluency, and unbroken sexual energy.

Kiss Classification

The French actress Mistinguette is famously quoted as saying "A kiss can be a comma, a question mark, or an exclamation point." Ah, how true, madame. The type of kiss you use on any given body part can greatly affect the way it feels to your man. One type

I like to kiss firmly—I hate really wet kisses—but my new boy-friend is a really sloppy kisser. It makes me not want to kiss him at all. Should I just break up with him?

♂ *Don:* I feel your pain. I remember one girl I kissed…once. It was like making out with a melting Jello mold. If you do like this guy, don't give up. When he kisses you sloppily, stop, smile, and whisper, "Kiss me hard." Do it every single time.

♀ *Debra:* If you can't find a way to let your boyfriend know exactly what you dislike about his technique, he'll go on thinking he's a kissing Casanova. Since you're still boyfriend-girlfriend, now's the time to establish good sexual communication. Talk about it. It may be the first sexual issue you have, but if you're destined to be together for a long time, it won't be the last.

of kiss might give him butterflies; the next might make him moan for more; and yet another might make him gasp. Moreover, certain types of kisses are suited to certain areas of the body. A French kiss on the mouth feels rapturous; a French kiss on the ear feels ridiculous (and is probably quite deafening).

The different types of kisses you may wish to use in a full-body kiss include the following.

THE FRENCH KISS This kiss is a deep, open-mouthed kiss in which lovers use their lips and tongues to arouse each other. A woman can suck on her man's tongue, use her tongue to circle and stroke his, and suck on or bite his lower lip. She can also trace her tongue along the inside of his lips, perhaps passing the frenulum (the thin flap of skin that connects the upper lip to the gum) with the tip of her tongue. The French kiss is perhaps the most intimate of all kisses, and for that reason there is a range of likes and dislikes. One man may be turned on by a lover grazing his teeth with her tongue, while another may find it unpleasant. The exchange of saliva that occurs during the French kiss makes it necessary for lovers to take brief breathers and swallow, lest the kiss turn from sexy to sloppy.

THE NIBBLE This kiss is simply a gentle bite. To maximize its pleasure, try leaving your lips in contact with your lover's skin while you nibble. Areas that respond best to nibbles include the lips, earlobes, and the nipples (if your man has sensitive nipples, that is). When nibbling his nipples, start out gently, and, if he likes it, let your nibbles get harder. Sometimes a brief flare of pain can inflame passion.

THE SUCK This kiss involves drawing an area of your man's body into your mouth with a sexy suction action. The earlobes, nipples, lips, and tongue all respond eagerly to sucking. Sucking a man's fingers and toes often leads to a powerfully quick wave of arousal because of the strong association with fellatio.

THE TONGUE SWIRL During this kiss, a woman uses the tip of her tongue to trace a small, wet circle on her man's skin. Tongue swirls feel particularly good on the neck, the area behind the ear, and the inner thigh. To vary the way this kiss feels to your lover, you can perform it with your lips pressed against his skin, or you can stick your tongue out of your mouth so that he only feels the tip touching his flesh.

THE LICK Anyone who's ever had an ice-cream cone knows how to perform the basics of this kiss. But there's more to the lick than polishing off a double scoop of the chocolate-fudge special. By changing the strength of your licks (gentle or aggressive), the length of body surface you cover (an inch or an entire inner thigh), and the shape of your tongue (pointed or flattened), you can affect the way a lick feels to your partner.

THE BUTTERFLY Typically, this oh-so-subtle kiss is performed by lovers fluttering their eyelashes together. But the eyelash flutter also feels good elsewhere, especially on those body spots that sport thinner skin, such as the inner arm or the back of the knee.

THE HOT TAMALE This is a spicy kiss that can be used on almost any body area with great effect. To perform it, inhale deeply, and then exhale in one long, slow, controlled breath. Keep your mouth very close to your man's body, and focus your exhalation on a small area of his skin. Your breath should be as hot and bothered as possible.

THE COOL FRONT This kiss is the chilly chaser to the hot tamale. The moment your hot tamale exhalation ends, pull your head back from your man's body, and, from a distance, blow a cool breath of fresh air onto the hot spot. This is a temperature change that'll really make him shiver.

THE ESKIMO KISS Kisses don't get any cuter than this northerly nose rub. Affectionate and playful, the Eskimo kiss is a wonderful way for your and your man's faces to be up close and personal without immediately falling into a French kiss. It's also a nice way to take a breather during a French-kissing marathon. You can follow your nose rubbing with either a quick, mischievous kiss on the end of your man's nose or a lingering, loving kiss on his forehead.

THE RIMMER The name of this kiss is derived from the sexual practice of analingus, aka rimming, which is the act of stimulating a lover's anus with one's mouth, particularly with the tongue.

The way you make first contact with the anal region is up to you and your man. The brave may jump in with long, steady licks over the anal sphincter that lead to confident tongue thrusts into the anus. The cautious may move slower, perhaps circling the anus with the tongue (rimming it) before experimentally pushing the tip of the tongue against the sphincter. Some men find even this slight pressure is enough to please.

In the same way that you can rim the anus by circling it with the tip of your tongue, you can rim other potentially erotic orifices of your man's body. These include the belly button, the ear flap and canal, and the mouth (specifically the surface and inside of the lips).

THE PENETRATOR This erotically invasive kiss could be called *tongue-fucking*. If performed in the anus, it's part and parcel of analingus, but, like the rimmer, the penetrator isn't limited to anal play. It can plunge its pleasure into any of your partner's bodily orifices, including the navel (for innies, at least), the ear canal, and the mouth.

THE FLICKER As if your tongue weren't tired enough, the flicker also puts it to work. This kiss scores high marks on the flirt-and-tease scale for its quick but electrifying touch. Just as you use your fingers to quickly flip a light switch, you use the tip of your tongue to flick over a part of your man's body and fire up his libido. The ear canal, nipples, navel, and anus all respond eagerly to the flicker's love-'em-and-leave-'em ways.

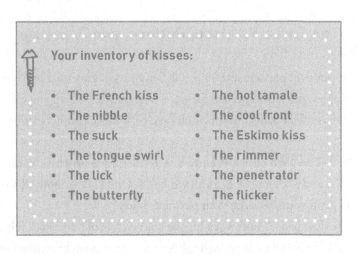

Your inventory of kisses:

- The French kiss
- The nibble
- The suck
- The tongue swirl
- The lick
- The butterfly

- The hot tamale
- The cool front
- The Eskimo kiss
- The rimmer
- The penetrator
- The flicker

The Whole Is Greater Than the Sum of Its Parts

Although a full-body kiss is comprised of a number of distinct kissing types, remember that the whole is greater than the sum of its parts. These kisses work best when they work together. The transition from one type of kiss to another—for example, from a tongue swirl on the neck to a flicker on a nipple—should be as smooth as silk.

Practice makes perfect, and it won't take you long to gain real proficiency in the art of full-body kissing. When this happens, you'll find that you naturally begin to expand your skills by combining the types of kisses outlined in this chapter to create your own trademark body kisses. Such is the unlimited passion and potential of the full-body kiss.

The Three Ps: Pace, Pattern, and Pressure

The physical performance of a full-body kiss is governed by three variables: pace, pattern, and pressure. These three Ps help you carry out the style of body kiss you've chosen, be it sweet, sinful, or sultry.

PACE The pace of a full-body kiss is the speed at which it proceeds, and is therefore determined by how quickly or how slowly you plant your kisses on your partner's body.

A slow pace is necessary for the sultry style of body kiss. This style is designed to be agonizingly erotic to your man by extending the seduction phase to heighten his sexual anticipation. The sultry style is also meant to showcase you as a skilled sexual vixen, a virtual Venus who takes her time and tortures her man with prolonged pleasure before treating him to release. Slow kisses that lustfully but languidly travel over his body will result in an intoxicatingly sultry full-body kiss.

A medium pace is best for the sweet style of body kiss. The sweet style is a very emotionally charged kiss, and a medium pace allows you to perform it at a steady speed, letting your man absorb the powerful emotions of the experience without being overwhelmed by an excruciatingly slow or exhaustingly fast pace. A medium pace is perhaps the most natural pace to use and is therefore great for body-kiss beginners.

A fast pace is ideal for the sinful style of body kiss. Nasty and desperate, a fast pace supports quickie blow jobs and naughty sexual role plays like Up Against a Wall. This pace is a lusty lightening strike that hits your partner's body fast and hard. It's all about the "physical" part of arousal and doesn't spend a lot of time rousing emotion or loitering in foreplay.

PATTERN Pattern is the flight path your kisses take as they move over your man's body, landing on his flesh according to schedule. Pattern is very dependent on the position of your partner's body as well as on whether he is fully, partially, or unclothed. A good knowledge of your man's erogenous zones is necessary to establish the most pleasurable pattern(s) your kisses should take, whether they move from head to toe, foot to forehead, or somewhere in between.

PRESSURE Pressure is the amount of force and/or compression with which your kisses fall on your lover's flesh. Changing the pressure of any given kiss or combination of kisses is a great way to increase your inventory of kissing types and to establish kissing style. For example, a feathery tongue swirl followed by a soft nibble is sweetly arousing; however, a strong tongue swirl followed by a hard nibble is sinfully ferocious. Kisses of different pressure can thus work alone and/or together to create an almost unlimited variety of full-body kissing experiences for your man.

Focusing on the three Ps of pace, pattern, and pressure will help you establish an overall rhythm to your full-body kiss, while simultaneously maintaining the spirit or style of kiss you've chosen. Learn to play these notes together, and you'll be able to conduct some truly beautiful music.

The one, two, threes of a body kiss:

(1) Choose a style: sweet, sinful, or sultry
(2) Use a variety of kissing types, from the French to the flicker
(3) Establish a flow through pace, pattern, and pressure

Body Blueprints

The "body blueprint" is the final product of all your study and skill. It is where everything you've learned about the art of full-body kissing comes together, enabling you to plan and perform this ultimate prelude to fellatio.

Essentially, a body blueprint is the mental flowchart you'll keep in mind as you perform the full-body kiss. It incorporates the style

How do you get a guy to enjoy foreplay, including body kissing, more? Mine always wants to fast-forward to orgasm.

♀ *Debra:* Change the way you and your partner think about sex, de-emphasizing the final destination—orgasm and ejaculation—and focusing instead on the journey. This approach is practiced by Tantric lovers, as they consider each moment of sexual togetherness to be orgasmic, not just the climax. If you and he can stop thinking of sex as a two-part deal (foreplay vs. orgasm, that is) you'll get a lot more out of your love life.

♂ *Don:* We once took in a starving stray puppy, and even years later he'd wolf down his food like it was his last meal. Sometimes guys feel the same way about sex. We really want to make sure we're going to get it. Reassure him that he is, and he'll relax enough to enjoy the appetizer.

of kiss you've chosen, the types of kisses you'll use, and the pace, pattern, and pressure with which you'll proceed. As you become more adept at body kissing, you'll find it progressively easier to create customized body blueprints to suit your man's unique pleasure preferences.

To begin, however, you may find it simpler to follow the sexy schematics we've drawn up. The following body blueprints are only modest examples of what is possible. So play the studious pupil and follow along to practice the art of full-body kissing; you'll graduate to master status before you know it.

Body Blueprint A

Position of partner: Sitting
Style: Sweet
Pace: Medium
Pattern: Circular
Pressure: Partner's usual preference
Types of kisses used: French, nibble, suck, Eskimo, lick, tongue
swirl, rimmer, penetrator

For several reasons, Body Blueprint A is a great one for beginners. First, it's actually a partial-body kiss rather than a full one, allowing you to dip your toes into the art of body kissing without jumping into the deep end on your first try. Second, it moves at a medium pace, which, as you'll remember, is the most natural and therefore easiest pace to use. Third, the pressure you'll use to deliver your kisses is also natural, being your partner's normal preference as opposed to a dramatically soft or hard pressure. And fourth, this body kiss is performed in the sweet style. How better to introduce this loving art into your sex life?

This partial-body kiss is most easily performed if your partner is fully unclothed. Choose a night when you and he are snuggling naked under the covers, perhaps watching a romantic movie in bed. To begin the body kiss, you can ask him to sit on the edge of the bed, and you can kneel on the floor in front of him. Better still, choose a quiet evening and ask him to share a bath with you. You can have him sit on the edge of the tub while you stay in the warmth of the water. A wet, naked woman is an arousing sight to a man, so seduce his body and his eyes by baring all.

Once your man is seated, kneel in front of him and ask him to kiss you. He'll have to lean down to reach your lips (which in itself is a sexy position for a man to kiss a woman). Meet his mouth softly, and then part your lips, caressing his lips with feathery kisses and teasing nibbles. Move into a deeper French kiss by gently sucking his tongue and brushing against it with your tongue. Remember that the very intimate nature of French-kissing makes it highly subjective. If your partner enjoys it, you can glide your tongue along the inside of his lips, lick along his teeth, brush your tongue against his, and explore the depths of his mouth.

Because this blueprint can be a bonding one, spend some time French-kissing your partner's mouth. Alternate your French kiss charges with Eskimo-kiss time-outs. This will give you time to swallow, but, just as important, it will also help maintain the sweet, romantic aura of this body kiss. When you're ready to continue, travel south by placing a line of soft kisses down your man's body from his Adam's apple to his navel.

Since the pattern of this partial-body kiss is circular, it will help if you can visualize a circle whose perimeter runs through your man's belly button, down over his hips, and across his thighs. His genitals are in the circle's center. Except for his genitals, which will have to wait until the chapter on fellatio for their fair share of affection, you will be kissing the area within the circle as well as its circumference.

Beginning at your man's belly button and moving in a clock-wise direction, plant a perimeter of simple kisses across his stom-ach, down his left side and hip, over the top of his thighs, and then up over his other hip and side, completing the circle at his navel. This not only outlines the area you'll be working in but also brings this area to erotic life by stimulating it and putting your man's senses on high alert.

If this is a bath-time body kiss, cup some warm water in your hands and shower his thighs, hips, and navel with water before your next series of kisses. It'll add a sexy wet warmth to the feel of your mouth. Bring your mouth to your man's navel and kiss it softly, then use the tip of your tongue to rim the outer edge of his belly button.

Again following the clockwise perimeter of the circle, move to his left side with one long lick, and stop over his hip to perform one or two tongue swirls. Place a path of kisses over the top of his thigh. Treat his left inner thigh to a single long lick, ending the lick with a tongue swirl at the top of his inner thigh. You should be dangerously close to but not touching his scrotum. Give his right inner thigh a similar long lick, also ending it with a tongue swirl.

Continue up your man's right hip and side in a progression of long and short licks, each interrupted by tongue swirls. Don't forget to keep your path slippery by gently splashing or spreading water over his skin. When you reach his navel, use the tip of your tongue to perform another rimmer, but follow this one by penetrating his belly button with your tongue and slowly wriggling it around inside the orifice.

You can continue to follow the circle in a clockwise direction as many times as you wish, drawing ever closer to his genitals to build his anticipation. Just keep in mind that the purpose of this exercise is to increase his arousal and to practice delayed gratification. Body kissing is fellatio foreplay, so keep your mouth off his manhood until it's time for oral sex.

Body Blueprint A at a glance:

- Have your man sit as you kneel between his legs.
- Begin with a French kiss, interrupted by Eskimo kisses.
- Kiss down his body to his navel.
- Place a circle of kisses across his belly, down one hip, over his thighs, and up his other hip.
- Rim his belly button.
- Retrace your circle of kisses, placing licks and tongue swirls on his inner thighs.
- Rim and penetrate his belly button with your tongue.
- Follow the circle again, drawing ever closer to his genitals.

BODY BLUEPRINT B

Position of partner: Supine
Style: Sultry
Pace: Slow
Pattern: Head to toe
Pressure: Light, average, and strong
Types of kisses used: French, nibble, suck, tongue swirl, lick, butterfly, hot tamale, cool front, Eskimo, rimmer, penetrator, flicker

Body Blueprint B lays the foundation for the quintessential full-body kiss. This one is a virtual cat bath that will have your man purring with delight. To begin, have your man lie naked on his back, staring up at the ceiling. This exposed position presents the best canvas on which to create this sultry-style, full-body–kiss masterpiece and to show your man what a sexual artist you are. It's best if he's lying comfortably on his bed, since he's in for a long session of slow-paced passion.

If you're playing out the Power Struggle fantasy, you can fasten your man's wrists to the headboard or, to achieve the same sense of erotic vulnerability, simply ask him to hang onto the headboard. With his arms overhead, the sides of his body—those large erogenous zones—are more accessible and more sensitive to the touch. Holding his hands at his sides, your fingers entwined in his, also lets him know that you're in control. This position, however, doesn't expose his sides as much, and it also monopolizes your hands when they could be of sexier use elsewhere.

The kissing pressure you'll use during this full-body kiss is variable: light pressure one moment, stronger the next; a hard suck or nibble on one area, then a soft suck or nibble on the next. The pattern you'll follow is head to toe, but this blueprint can work just as well from the ground up. As long as you cover every inch of his body in sequence—again, with the exception of those "special inches," which are dealt with in chapter 8—you're on the right track.

Begin by placing a soft, welcoming kiss on your man's forehead. Next, slowly move your face close to his and give him an intimate Eskimo kiss, letting your noses rub for several long moments before, ever so suggestively moving your nose to his ear. Nuzzle his ear with your nose, and then, again with slow, seductive speed, breathe into his ear. Let the tip of your tongue touch the opening to his ear canal. Linger there for several moments before rimming it. Slide the tip of your tongue into his ear canal, penetrating it. As you withdraw your tongue, take his earlobe into your mouth for a nibble. Move into a tongue swirl on the area behind his earlobe.

When you're finished with that ear, brush your face against his cheek as you move your mouth to meet his lips. French-kiss him slowly and gently at first, then let your mounting desire show as you kiss him with desperate, deep kisses. Explore his mouth, suck on his tongue, and suck and nibble his lower lip. Again, brush your face against his as you move to his other ear. Repeat the same sequence of rimmers, penetrators, nibbles, and tongue swirls on this ear.

Move at a lustful but leisurely pace down the side of his neck, treating this ultrasensitive area to a series of light kisses, licks, and tongue swirls. Keep your lips against your man's skin as you plant eager tongue swirls, so that you're French-kissing his neck. Slide your kisses to his Adam's apple. Circle it with your tongue, suck it, and travel up the other side of his neck with a bevy of light kisses, licks, and tongue swirls.

Although your mouth is the star player in a full-body kiss, your hands are great costars. Use them in a supporting capacity by gliding your fingers over an area of your man's body, stimulating his skin and making it anxious for your mouth. If your man's arms are over his head, graze both of his inner arms with your fingertips, first upward and then back down. Lean over and give him a barely-there butterfly kiss on the inner elbow of one arm. Move to the other inner elbow to perform a hot tamale, quickly followed by a cool front.

Next, slowly travel down your man's chest with alternating long and short licks, some too hard, others too soft. Take turns flicking each nipple with the tip of your tongue before gently nibbling, then biting, and finally sucking them. Don't rush it. Take your time as you tease his nipples.

Plant a row of kisses down the centerline of your man's body until you reach his navel. Before kissing it, drag your fingertips down the sides of his body, raising goose pimples of pleasure along this sexy stretch of skin. Lean over and place a number of tongue swirls, flicks, licks, even nibbles along this length. A hot tamale, with or without a cool front in tow, would also work well here.

Once again, remember to keep your speed in check as you travel south. You might be feeling more eager, but set your libido on cruise and maintain an excruciatingly slow mph, even as your desire—and your man—tempt you to pick up the pace on the downhill stretch.

Move from your man's side to his belly button in one long lick. Rim the opening and then penetrate it with your tongue. If he's an "outie," flick the button with the tip of your tongue, and then suck it.

When his navel's had enough, lick him downward, to where his pubic hair starts. Carry the lick over his hip. As you did with his inner arms and his sides, glide your fingertips along his inner thighs to prep them for your kisses. Tongue swirls and nibbles to the inner thighs will result in a strong groin ache, so don't cave if he tries to coax you toward his genitals. Stand your ground, and gently suck on the skin of his upper inner thigh.

If you really want to spike his mental arousal while giving yourself a thrill, straddle your man's body backward so that you're facing his feet. Let him look up to admire your bare bum and back. Lean forward to let your breasts press against his groin as you continue to kiss his thighs. To fire up his arousal, masturbate yourself by grinding your clitoris against his body. Make a long show of this homemade XXX feature. After all, you're the pro.

When you're ready for the next scene, snake down your partner's body and legs, leaving a trail of licks in your wake as you reach the end of this sultry full-body kiss. Suck on his toes, and, to make sure he catches the reference, tell him you can't wait to suck his cock.

Body Blueprint B at a glance:

- Have your man lie down, and then place a welcoming kiss on his forehead.
- Kiss his ear area and his mouth.
- Place kisses, licks, and tongue swirls on his neck.
- Graze his inner arms with your fingertips, and kiss his inner elbows.
- Move down his chest, licking his chest and tongue-flicking his nipples.
- Kiss down to his navel, kissing and grazing his sides with your fingertips.
- Lick down to his pubic hair.
- Graze his inner thighs with your fingertips, and then kiss them.
- Straddle him backward, and lean over to press your breasts into his groin.
- Snake down his body and legs, licking them, and suck his toes.

Body Blueprint C

Position of partner: Standing
Style: Sinful
Pace: Fast
Pattern: Repeating, up and down
Pressure: Strong
Types of kisses used: French, tongue swirl, lick, nibble, suck,
   hot tamale, cool front, flicker

Body Blueprint C is one for the she-devils among us. It is a fast-paced, nasty, aggressive body kiss with rough-and-tumble contact that, while seeming random and frantic, actually follows a planned pattern. To start this sinful full-body kiss, catch your clothed man off guard and assertively push him against a wall. For best effect, make it a wall outside the bedroom (providing the kids are at Grandma's and the curtains are closed, of course). Since this body kiss is full of raw energy, push him hard and don't worry if your mother-in-law's picture falls off the wall; you can pick it up later.

Press your body against your man's and initiate a desperate, deep French kiss. Suck and bite his lower lip, then suck his tongue. Clutch at his clothing as you kiss him. Struggle to slip your hands up his shirt and down his pants. Take a step back and undress yourself, ordering him to do the same. Remember that this is a bad-girl body kiss, so don't water it down with modesty. Save the good-girl act for the sweet style.

When you're both undressed, roughly spin your man around so that he's facing the wall, his body pressed against it. You now have access to the back of his neck, his back, his buttocks, and the backs of his legs. These are the areas you may normally neglect in favor of his frontal parts.

Attack the nape of his neck with a hard, wet tongue swirl. Quickly move down to his lower back and place a similar tongue swirl there. Lick along his spine, moving upward, all the way from his tailbone to the nape of his neck. Nibble the sides of his neck and his shoulders hard, as if you don't recognize the difference between passion and pain!

Travel back down your man's spine with a series of short licks. Holding on to his hips for support, smother his lower back and buttocks with a frenzy of hot kisses, tongue swirls, and nibbles. Continue down the backs of his legs, alternating your kisses from one to the other, until you reach the back of his knees. Nibble the back of one knee. Do a hot tamale/cool front combo on the other.

Move back up his body in one swift motion, only letting your tongue flick over his flesh a few times. When you're standing again, spin him around and push his back against the wall. Attack his neck (especially the area of his Adam's apple) with a tongue swirl and suck.

Without missing a beat, grab on to your guy's hips for balance and lower your body until your mouth is level with his groin. Kiss the sensitive crease where his leg meets his hip, thoroughly washing this erotic area with a flood of tongue swirls, licks, hot tamales, nibbles, and flickers. Don't forget to wash the other side, too.

Change channels midshow by unexpectedly returning to his upper body. Flick his nipples with your tongue, and nibble them with as much force as he can take. You're forgiven if you press your body against his genitals; just keep your kisser clear, at least for a while longer.

Drop to your knees. Lick his inner thighs for a brief moment. Stop, and take one of his hands in yours. Suck his middle finger as you look up at him. Keep sucking his finger, but shift your eyes to gaze hungrily at his erection. Moan loudly, as if his manhood is driving you crazy with desire. You can even touch yourself as you continue to suck his finger. Whew! What man could ask for better foreplay to fellatio?

Body Blueprint C at a glance:

- While standing, begin with a deep, desperate French kiss on his mouth.
- Undress, and spin his body around, pressing it against the wall.
- Aggressively kiss his nape, and then kiss along his spine, down and back up.
- Lick down his spine again, covering his buttocks with a frenzy of kisses.
- Kiss down the back of his legs.
- Kiss back up his body, and spin him around, pressing his back against the wall.
- Kiss his neck and Adam's apple.
- Holding onto his hips, kiss his groin area (*not* his genitals).
- Move upward, tongue-flicking his nipples.
- Drop to your knees, and suck his finger while admiring his erection.

BODY BLUEPRINT D

Position of partner: On hands and knees
Style: Sultry
Pace: Slow
Pattern: Circular
Pressure: Comfortable
Types of kisses used: tongue swirl, nibble, lick, flicker, rimmer, penetrator

In Body Blueprint D, the *D* stands for *doggy*—doggy position, that is. But why bottom up, you ask? Because this blueprint details a partial-body kiss that focuses on the buttocks, hips, backs of the thighs, and the anus and that includes analingus.

While analingus and anal play are a large part of many heterosexual couples' sex lives, not all couples have ventured into this touchy territory. For many straight men, anal play is a definite no-no. For other straight men, anal play is a definite... *maybe*. It's for those brave souls that this backdoor blueprint is designed.

To make a man's derrière deflowering as stress free as possible, this partial-body kiss is performed in the sultry style, at a slow, I-won't-make-any-sudden-moves pace. You'll also use a comfortable level of pressure. Translation: You'll go as soft, or as hard, as your man instructs. Unlike other body blueprints, he's in complete control. Even if his face is buried in the pillow, he's calling the shots. If you want your man to remain receptive to anal play, he has to trust you implicitly and know that you won't do anything unwanted or unexpected. So while there's nothing wrong with gently urging him on, make sure you immediately hit the brakes if he says "stop."

💜 *A caveat about analingus:* It may be sexy, but it isn't always safe. At the least, a shower is essential to ensure good anal hygiene. If there are *any* risk factors associated with you and your partner performing this activity, including but not limited to the presence or possibility of STDs, hepatitis, or intestinal parasites, use a barrier over the anus (like a dental dam, a condom that's been slit open, or even plastic food wrap), or simply find your fun elsewhere. A barrier should be used if you're going from analingus to fellatio.

Now that the warnings are out of the way, let's get back to the action. Ask your man to get onto all fours on the bed, and then squat behind him. For the best possible access, have him rest on his elbows so that his bum sticks up in the air.

Cast your memory back to Body Blueprint A. Remember the circle you visualized in that partial-body kiss (where your man's genitals were in the circle's center)? You're going to visualize a similar circle in Body Blueprint D. In fact, you can consider it the flip side of Blueprint A. When your man is on his hands and knees, the circle arcs over his lower back, down one hip, across the back of his upper thighs, and then runs up the other hip to return to his lower back. His buttocks should fill most of the circle's area, and his anus should be bull's-eye center.

Just as you worked in a circular pattern in Blueprint A, so, too, will you follow a clockwise circular scheme in Blueprint D. Think of yourself as a vulturelike vixen, circling your prey with patience and skill until you're ready to zoom in for the kill. To begin, caress your man's buttocks with your hands, perhaps delivering a tender love slap to his behind, just to get his blood flowing. Explore the area of your circle with your hands. Run your palms over his hips and across the back of his legs. Knead his buttocks gently, separating them slightly to let your thumbs lightly graze his anus.

Next, kiss your man's lower back with a soft tongue swirl so that he can feel the warmth of your mouth on his skin. Traveling clockwise, leave a trail of soft kisses over his right hip. When you reach the back of his leg, change from soft kisses to gentle tongue flicks and nibbles. Carry these tongue flicks and nibbles to the back of his left leg. Leave soft kisses up over his left hip, and return to the start line on his lower back.

Repeat this circling-in pattern, drawing ever closer to his anus with each pass, until your partner is primed for analingus. To keep each circle fresh and exciting, change the pressure with which you perform the different types of kisses.

Separate your partner's buttocks to expose his anus. Ask his permission to kiss it. When he says yes, place soft, no-frills kisses on his anus. Stop, and ask him if you can do more. When you have the go-ahead, kiss his anus again. This time, stick your tongue out, and begin to lightly rim his anus. Stop. Again, ask for permission to proceed. When you have it, lick his anus with a flattened tongue.

This initial series of kisses, rimmers, and licks should be performed at a slow pace in a reassuringly predictable pattern and with only light pressure. Pause at regular intervals to tell him how much you enjoy experimenting with him in this way, and how turned on the experience is making you. This will give him confidence while simultaneously giving him time to absorb what is happening. Anal-region regulars may not require this kind of TLC, but newbies need it.

If your guy is game to go further, spread his buttocks apart and spend a few moments rimming his anus. Press your tongue against his anus. Apply gentle pressure, letting the tip penetrate the sphincter. You can push your tongue in as far as you and/or he are comfortable with. He may enjoy the feeling of your tongue wriggling around just inside his anus. He may also experience pleasure from your tongue thrusting in and out of his anus, penetrating him with a regular, rhythmic motion.

Body Blueprint D at a glance:

- Have your man get onto all fours.
- Caress and love-slap his buttocks.
- Run your hands over his hips and across the back of his legs.
- Knead his buttocks, separating them and gently grazing his anus.
- Kiss his lower back.
- Place a circle of kisses down one hip, across the back of his legs, and up the other hip.
- Retrace the circle, drawing ever closer to his anus.
- Separate his buttocks and kiss his anus, rimming and penetrating it with your tongue.

The Best-Laid Plans

Having a body blueprint is essential when embarking on a full- or even partial-body kiss. Not having one is like going grocery shopping without a list: You end up wandering the aisles, wasting time, and forgetting half the items you need to buy. Therefore, to make sure that you get the job done with efficiency and skill, always plan your body kiss in advance.

While the sample blueprints we've included are good teaching tools, they're not right for everyone. Even the best-laid plans sometimes need revising to avoid going awry, and we won't take it personally if you choose to use these blueprints as general guidelines rather than carved-in-stone schematics. For example, you can mix and match the types of kisses you use or adjust the pace, pattern, and/or pressure for even more variety. You can even experiment with performing each blueprint in a different style. In the end, the plan is yours to lay.

A Kiss Isn't Just a Kiss

A full-body kiss isn't just a kiss; it's also a bonding experience, a way to learn about your lover's body, an exciting way to spice up a sex life, and a mouthwatering appetizer for the main course—fellatio. Full-body kissing is an art, not a science, so expand your erotic creativity and stretch your sexual imagination to keep the passion of this very special practice alive in your love life.

5 : The Skin-Tingling Treatment

Once you've mastered the basics of full-body kissing, you may want to practice more advanced techniques to keep your body kisses exciting and new. An easy way to do this is to add more physical sensations to the overall experience. You can do this in any number of ways, as long as the sensation is one that complements and enhances the feel of the full-body kiss and doesn't distract from or overwhelm it.

For example, drizzling chocolate body paint on your man's lower back and licking it off is sexy. Pouring corn syrup down his leg and licking it off is sticky. It also leaves behind a gluey sweet trail that breaks the smooth flow needed during a body kiss. Happily for those who don't like to mix sex with supper, food isn't the only way to spice up a body kiss. Experimenting with different textures is also a great way to add that extra touch to your lip service.

You Scratch My Back...

Taylor and Michelle, together for six years, can testify to the thrill that texture can bring to the body kiss. "We always shower together before sex," says Taylor. "We use the time as foreplay by kissing and fondling each other. We do a lot of body kissing where we take turns on each other. Sometimes we get into oral and finish each other off in the shower, but usually we head into the bedroom."

"We're kind of predictable," adds Michelle. "That's not really a bad thing, because we're both happy with our game routine. But I wanted to throw Taylor a curve ball. Just to remind him that I still could."

So what kind of curve ball did Michelle throw?

"A back scratcher," Taylor reveals. "It was nothing special, just an old, cracked, back scratcher that had been sitting on the side of the tub for months. Who would've thought it had such hidden talents?"

"Taylor had his back to me in the shower," says Michelle. "The water was running down his back, and I was kissing up and down his spine. I know how much he likes that, so I always do it the same way, every single time. But this time I caught sight of the back scratcher out of the corner of my eye. It was just lying there, minding its own business, and I suddenly had the idea of using it to scratch his back for him."

"I was enjoying Michelle's kisses on my back," Taylor continues. "She always follows the same pattern—up and down, maybe a few kisses over a shoulder blade—but I like it. Her kisses went up to my neck and I expected them to move back down again, but instead I felt a light grazing sensation run down my backbone. Her kisses followed a moment later, kind of trailing behind the scratch. I felt the difference right away."

"I did this whole new zigzag pattern on his back," says Michelle. "Back and forth, then around in a circle, and then zigzag again. I stopped now and then to kiss a spot somewhere on his back. Then I'd use the scratcher again. Sometimes I'd scratch hard; other times I'd scratch so lightly that he could hardly feel it. He really responded to it; and I felt sexier just doing something different."

"I don't usually get a strong erection in the shower unless we're really into oral," says Taylor, "but the raking sensation all over my back made me hard. The combination of scratches and kisses gave me a good erection. I was anxious for her to finish me off."

"It turned me on to see Taylor so eager," says Michelle, "not that he doesn't usually have good response, but it's nice to see I can still get him turbocharged once in a while."

Back to the Blueprint

Indeed, the shower and bath can play host to a plethora of skin-tingling textures that you can incorporate into your body kiss. Recall Body Blueprint A from the last chapter, which had your man sitting on the edge of the bathtub while you, immersed in the water like a naughty sea nymph, performed a partial-body kiss on him. Although Blueprint A suggested you splash water on his skin to enhance the feel of your kisses, you can create even more waves by first using a textured product on him.

A loofah is perhaps the best textured bath product to use. Soap it up, and then massage your man's hips and thighs, especially his inner thighs, in small circles that complement the circular pattern of the body kiss. The natural exfoliating action of the loofah will stimulate sensation in this area, sending a flow of arousal to his groin.

If you don't want anything to come between you and your man, use an exfoliating cream/scrub or body polish that you can rub into his skin with your hands. Many men love to be washed by a woman; it's sweetly sexy. And since Body Blueprint A is in the sweet style, it's the perfect way to lather up his libido.

Fun with Fur

The slow, sultry full-body kiss outlined in Body Blueprint B also provides an opportunity to bring extra tingle and texture to body kissing. Its indulgent approach facilitates the use of various texture tools, one of which is fur. Sensual fur massage is practiced by many couples and is a decadent way to seductively soothe your man. You can purchase a fur mitten that is specifically made for sensual massage. There is a good variety of these available, each made with a different type of fur to achieve a unique feel. (On a humane note, please consider choosing faux fur out of kindness to our minx, bunny, and fox friends.)

To improvise, ransack your kid's room, and hijack one of his or her softer stuffed toys. An old, eyeless, teddy bear amputee with the stuffing coming out of its neck may not look as sexy as a designer fur glove, but it'll still elicit a respectable level of sensory stimulation if used properly. If you have long hair, you can also use your own mane to brush your man's body with soft sensuality. The fur (or hair) massage should follow the same head-to-toe pattern as the full-body kiss.

To enrich the sensation of your kisses, stimulate your man's bare skin with such textured tools as a wet or dry loofah, an exfoliating scrub, your hair, or a fur mitten.

To switch sensations, drip-dry the loofah from Body Blueprint A, and use its dry, scratchy surface to bring your partner's skin to life. Lightly polish his entire body with it, again following the same head-to-toe pattern as that for the fur massage and/or full-body kiss. Be sure to pay attention to the sides of his body, particularly if his arms are over his head and his sides are exposed. This full-body scratch is a great follow-up to a fur massage—he might be itchy!

Erotic Massage

The enrapturing stroke of a sensual massage is another sensation that can bring skin-tingling eroticism to your man's full-body–kiss experience, particularly if it's an all-nighter like the body kiss in Blueprint B. In the same way that full-body kissing is a bonding exercise, the passionate, prolonged intimacy of erotic massage can strengthen an emotional and physical bridge between lovers, not to mention the effect it has on the libido!

The popularity of sensual massage has spawned a huge array of products with which to bathe your man's body in pure, unadulterated pleasure. Massage oils are available in an almost endless selection of scents—from nice and natural to fruity and fragrant—and consistencies, from honey thick to milky thin. Sensual massage creams and lotions are just as effective as oils and are available in at least as wide a selection. Some massage products are flavored (not always deliciously so); others have a wonderful warming sensation when rubbed into the skin; and still others pull double-duty as lubricants.

Erotic massage is a natural form of touch between lovers. Unlike therapeutic massage, there's no right or wrong way to caress your man. There's only one rule: If it feels good, do it. Then do it again. That being said, it may be helpful to have an advance idea of where and how you're going to massage him.

This is a simple step-by-step sample of a sensual massage. It follows a general head-to-toe pattern:

Step 1: Set the mood (lower the lighting, raise the temperature, unplug the phone), prepare your bedroom and bed (lock the door for privacy, spread an older sheet or towels over the bed to avoid staining your linen), and gather your supplies (two rolled towels, a hand towel, and your massage oil/lotion/cream of choice).

Step 2: Have your naked man lie facedown on the bed. Place a rolled towel under his collarbones to raise his shoulders off the bed. This will let him rest his forehead on the bed and keep his head straight. To support the lower back, place another rolled towel under his ankles.

Step 3: Place your fingertips on your partner's head and rake them over his scalp, along the back of his neck, down his back (one hand on each side of his spine), and over his buttocks. Make like a cat and sheath your nails, lightly raking with your finger pads only. Beginning at his shoulders, rake down both arms, then down the back of both legs.

Step 4: Return to your partner's head. Massage his scalp as if treating him to a deep scalp-stimulating shampooing.

Step 5: Warm the massage oil between your hands. Spread it across your man's back in long gliding strokes, then over his neck and shoulders. Smooth it down each arm, and down each leg. Use generous amounts of oil, and apply with firm but not forceful strokes.

Step 5: Knead your partner's shoulders with well-oiled hands. Use the lubrication of the oil to slide your hands down his arms to his wrists. When you reach his hands, use your thumbs to stroke his palms.

Step 6: Warm more oil in your hands. With open fingers, run your flattened hands down your man's back, on either side of his spine. Continue over his lower back, but be careful not to put too much pressure on his lower back. Keeping your hands in the same open-fingered position, slide your hands up his back, again on either side of his spine. Your fingers should point the way, whether you're moving up or down his back.

Step 7: Starting at the top of his backbone, put the fingers of one hand in the V shape of the peace sign, and straddle his spine with your index and middle fingers. Move the V down and then up the sides of his spine, using as much pressure as he likes, being careful to avoid putting direct pressure on the backbone itself.

Step 8: Using an ample amount of oil, place your flattened hands over his shoulder blades and fan your hands outward in opposite directions, stroking with the heels of your hands. Move your hands down a few inches and place them on either side of his spine. Again, fan your hands out in opposite directions, all the way across his back and down both sides. Repeat this all the way to his lower back.

Step 9: Glide your flattened hands up his back. Make circular strokes over the entire surface of his back.

Step 10: Knead his shoulders again, using a love or "lobster" pinch to squeeze and lift the muscle.

Step 11: Drag your fingers down the sides of his neck. Put your fingers in a stiff rake formation: Rake his back downward over his buttocks until you reach his legs.

Step 12: Flatten your hands, and, again using the massage oil as lubrication, slide your hands down the back of both legs without using too much pressure.

Step 13: Lift each foot in turn and thumb-stroke the soles (do this the same way that you thumb-stroked the palms of his hands). Rotate each ankle in slow circles.

And now for the flip side . . .

Step 14: Have your man lie on his back. Place one of the rolled towels under his neck, the other under the backs of his knees.

Step 15: Place your thumbs in the middle of your man's forehead.

Gently sweep outward, into his hairline. Position your thumbs on the inside edges of his eyebrows, and again stroke outward from the midline. Gently massage his temples with your fingertips. Pull his earlobes gently. Sweep your thumbs over his cheekbones.

Step 16: Warm the massage oil between your hands. Spread it over your partner's shoulders, letting your hands glide all the way down his arms. Lift each hand in turn, first pressing your thumb into the palm, and then squeezing each finger with a milking motion. Rotate each wrist in turn.

Step 17: Using more massage oil, move down your man's chest—commenting on his strength and masculinity, of course!— and do a series of well-lubed, clockwise, circular strokes over his belly.

Step 18: Avoiding contact with his genitals, glide your hands down over his hips. Without applying too much pressure, run your flattened hands down both of his legs.

Step 19: Massage each foot in turn with deep thumb strokes. Lace your fingers between his toes. Pull gently on each toe.

Step 20: Return to your man's head. Using just your fingertips, rake down his body from head to toe with feathery strokes.

Finis!

An erotic massage is an arousing experience. It can, however, also have a sedative effect, particularly since your man hasn't yet had direct genital stimulation to keep him awake. To prevent the mood turning from sexy to slumber, ask your man to stretch several times during the massage. He should do invigorating full-body stretches, with his arms over his head, holding each stretch for about ten seconds.

Erotic massage moves at a glance:

- The rake: Over the scalp, back, buttocks, and down arms and legs
- The glide: Across the back and shoulders, and down arms and legs
- The knead: For shoulders
- The thumb stroke: For palms and soles
- The V stroke: For either side of the spine
- The outward fan: For the back
- The circular stroke: For the back and belly
- The sweep: For the forehead and cheekbones

Sensory Delights and Lip Service

While you can use the different textural sensations of fur, loofah, and erotic body massage in different orders (just don't use fur after you've used an oily massage product), we recommend a soft-scratchy-soothing sequence to best exploit contrasting sensory effects. You are, however, the best judge of what gets your guy's juices flowing, so keep your own counsel.

Also, it isn't necessary to employ all of these textures or sensations in one session. The last thing you want to do is rush through a body kiss so that you can cram everything in. If time is of the essence, choose only one erotic extra.

It's your call whether you perform an entire fur and/or loofah and/or massage treatment before or after a full-body kiss, or whether you interrupt the flow of your body kiss to supplement it with these added sensations. We recommend using these or other erotic extras either before the body kiss begins or after it ends; this ensures an unbroken rhythm while allowing your man to bask in one sensory delight at a time.

Remember that full-body kissing is about using your mouth as a sexual organ. Other sensations are secondary and should never distract from the services your lips are providing.

What the Devil?

Now that we've added a few sweet and sultry extras to the body kiss, let's start thinking dirty and do something more sinful. The rough-and-tumble, up-against-a-wall sex struggle of Body Blueprint C gives us a great excuse to get a little nasty. The items you can use to add sinful sensations to your man's body kiss are many. Your choice depends on how naughty your inner she-devil is feeling.

While *Lip Service* doesn't cover fetish or BDSM material, we'd be remiss in our duties if we didn't suggest a little slap and tickle. And where better to bring out the leather than during a sinful body

During a sinful body kiss, use mild BDSM toys— including whips, paddles, and ticklers—to add pain and pleasure to your lip service.

kiss? Flogging toys—such as whips, crops, paddles, and canes—can really help you assert your sexual authority, while feather ticklers can help heal the pain.

When your man is pushed against the wall, with his back to you, you can alternate your soft touches with the sharp edges these toys can deliver. It's a devilishly delicious contrast. Try a tickle to the buttocks, followed by a stinging slap, followed by a healing tongue-swirl kiss to soothe the sore spot. Despite the rough treatment, or perhaps because of it, your man will be a willing victim.

But you don't have to dive into the world of whips and chains to be nasty. Ten of the sexiest, sauciest sex tools on the market are at your fingertips—literally. A woman's fingernails can do more than look good. They can also leave a path of pleasure behind them. Paint your fingernails blood red and drag them down your man's back like a minx in heat. When it comes to sex, pain and pleasure are often indistinguishable.

Feel the Burn

Body Blueprint D—your man's analingus adventure—offers another chance to skim the surface of BDSM, but don't introduce this element into anal kissing until you've been playing in the backyard for a while.

Spanking, whether you use your hand or some kind of paddle, brings a burn to the buttocks that some people find heightens stimulation in this area. It can also increase overall arousal. Start with gentle love pats and work your way up to a playfully punishing spank.

Hot-wax play is a practice where lovers drip candle wax on each other's bare skin. This results in a high-temperature erotic sensation that can be strikingly intense. Wax-play enthusiasts claim there's nothing like it, whether you're the dripper or the drippee, since the act itself is so sexually charged. How better to bring burning desire to the bedroom?

 Want it even hotter? Spanking and wax play can bring a sexy burn into your bedroom.

♥ Wax play warrants a capitalized CAVEAT. This is a practice that requires some study before lighting up. If you wish to experiment with wax play, visit a sex shop and purchase a sex candling kit. These are also available online. A specialty wax kit will contain the proper type of candle (low heat, raw paraffin, no additives) and may also come with instructions and/or warnings. Using an improper candle (including beeswax, votive, and tapered) can result in serious burns and/or skin irritation, so don't risk it.

Does This Match?

Adding extra physical sensations to a body kiss, be it texture, temperature, or sensual touch, can enhance the pleasure of your mouth moves. Just make sure the erotic extra you choose matches the mood you've set as well as the style of body kiss you're performing. For example, dragging an ice cube down your lover's back just after a soothing massage stroke will have him jumping off the bed, not moaning in ecstasy. A soft, slow, gentle scratch would feel far sexier.

Before you add that special something to your lip service, put yourself in your partner's place by asking yourself two questions. First, what kind of physical response will the added stimulus elicit? Second, what kind of mental response will it generate? If the answers to these questions are positive, it's a good bet that your erotic extra(s) will go well with your full-body kiss.

6 : His Parts

S o, you're just dying to discover the whereabouts of the bulbo-cavernous artery and the corpus spongiosum? Your life won't be complete until you have a thorough understanding of the seminal vesicles? Forgive us, but we don't intend to bombard you with a textbook collection of cross-section diagrams featuring the anatomical wonders of the male sexual organs. Nor do we intend to dive into detailed expositions on the inner and outer workings of such. The information is out there if you want it. As you'll see, *Lip Service* takes a less academic, more hands-on approach to helping you learn about your particular man's particulars.

Taking Matters into Your Own Hands

The next time your man has an erection, stop what you're doing (he'll think you're going for delayed gratification!) and look at his genitals. *Really* look at them. Take his genitals in your hands and examine their different shapes, surfaces, bumps, ridges, and nooks and crannies. Notice the length, width, and texture of his shaft as well as the shape and smoothness of the head. If he's uncircumcised, notice how his foreskin looks and feels as you draw it down his penis. Feel the wrinkly skin of his scrotum, and see how it hangs in relation to his penis. Squeeze it gently, noting the way his testicles feel and move inside. Now run your fingers through his pubic hair. Is it thick or trimmed? Or perhaps he removes it completely.

Of course you've seen your guy's genitals many times. But have you ever stopped to really examine these special parts of his body? If not, it's time to take matters into your own hands and to discover the most erogenous spots on his genitals. It's the only way to learn precisely what makes them, and him, tick.

Pleasure Island

A man's groin area is an island of pleasure that sets it apart from the rest of his body. And what do you do on an island? That's right, you look for treasure. It's time to play pirate and find the riches that lay just beneath the surface of your man's private Pleasure Island. This lushly erogenous location boasts a treasure trove of feel-good gold, but where to look for it? Happily, your quest is an easy one since, as they say in the pirate movies, X marks the spot. Find your man's X-spots, and you'll make him wealthier than if you'd found a buried chest of gold doubloons.

X Marks the Spot

Your man's X-spots include the following:

THE GLANS This is the head of the penis. This "mushroom cap" is a hotbed of nerve endings and is highly sensitive to stimulation. The glans is covered by the foreskin in uncircumcised (uncut) men, making its grand appearance when the penis is erect.

THE CORONAL RIDGE The coronal ridge (or corona) is the rim that runs around the glans or head of the penis, separating it from the shaft of the penis. Like the glans, it is very responsive to erotic stimulation.

THE FRENULUM In circumcised (cut) men, the frenulum is an erogenous, V-shaped spot on the underside of the penis, where the head meets the shaft. Some men may find it very sensitive, others less so. Some men have a more pronounced flap of a frenulum, particularly if they've been circumcised as an adult and the frenulum was not removed. In uncircumcised men, the frenulum connects the foreskin to the shaft. For better or for worse, we tend to use this term in a broad sense to refer to the general area or tissue on the underside of the penis, again where the head meets the shaft.

THE SHAFT The shaft of the penis is the smooth "rod" that extends from the head to the base. It is not as richly endowed with nerve endings as the glans, coronal ridge, or frenulum, but sexual strokes, including those with the mouth, feel fantastic. Some men find that the satiny-smooth underside of their shaft is particularly sensitive. In uncircumcised men, the shaft is covered with the foreskin.

THE BASE This is simply the bottom of the shaft. The base of the penis is a very useful part: For example, you can grip it to keep your man's erection steady while you perform fellatio, or you can slide a penis ring around it to help him last longer (penis rings will be discussed in chapter 9).

THE PUBIC HAIR Depending on your guy's coloring, ethnicity, and personal fuzziness factor, his pubic hair might be coarse or fine, thick or thin, sparse or abundant, curly or straight, dark or light. It may be localized around his genitals, or it may spread up to his abdomen, down to his thighs. The way your man keeps his pubic hair—whether au naturale, trimmed, or shaved—is something you and he should both be happy with. Running your fingers through your man's pubic hair and/or gently tugging it can feel good during fellatio; however, some basic hair care is necessary to avoid getting those distracting hairs in your mouth.

THE SCROTAL SAC This is the thin, wrinkly pouch underneath the penis. The scrotal sac (or scrotum) contains the testicles. Generally, when a man is very aroused (or it's cold out!) the scrotum contracts to become high and tight. When he is not aroused (or it's a hot summer day), the scrotum hangs lower and looser. The skin on the scrotum is sensitive to touch and shouldn't be forgotten during fellatio. For example, some men enjoy having their scrotum gently pulled, squeezed, and/or bounced in their lover's hands.

THE TESTICLES The testicles, known affectionately as the "balls," are the two oval-shaped organs that are housed inside the scrotal sac. Many men find gentle manipulation of the testicles to be very pleasurable, and, as with the scrotum, a woman should remember to incorporate testicle stimulation into fellatio.

THE PERINEUM Located behind the scrotum, between it and the anus, is a very sensitive erogenous zone called the perineum. This small stretch of skin is loaded with nerve endings. Touching, stroking, and/or massaging the perineum can feel very good. Applying pressure to this area during sexual activity, such as pressing your fingers or knuckles against it, may stimulate the prostate gland. Many men find this sensation highly orgasmic.

THE ANUS The anus and rectum are inundated with nerve endings and therefore have incredible pleasure potential. Whether they are stimulated via analingus or anal penetration, involving the anus and rectum in sexual activity, including fellatio, can bring a whole new level of excitement to a couple's sex life.

THE PROSTATE Talk about buried treasure! The prostate gland is located inside a man's body, under the bladder, in front of the rectum. Since the nerves that control a man's erection are attached to the prostate, this walnut-size wonder can deliver whale-size pleasure. The prostate gland is sometimes referred to as the male G-spot and, when stimulated, it can greatly intensify the strength and ecstasy of an orgasm. (Stimulation of the prostate will be covered in chapter 8.)

Your man's X-spots at a glance:

- The glans
- The coronal ridge
- The frenulum
- The shaft
- The base
- The pubic hair
- The scrotal sac and the testicles
- The perineum
- The anus
- The prostate

The Whole Is Greater Than the Sum of Its Parts

The next time you're intimate with your man, look at his genitals. What do you see? Hopefully after reading this chapter, you'll see more than just a "cock and balls." Instead, we hope you notice, and then take the time to visit, the individual erogenous zones of Pleasure Island, including the glans and coronal ridge, the frenulum, the satiny underside of the shaft, the scrotum, and the other X-spots that grace your guy's genitals. By stimulating each of his individual parts, you exponentially increase his pleasure as a whole.

7 : His Passion

Okay. We've convinced you that the mouth is a sexual organ. You've studied male erogenous zones, mastered the arts of dirty talk and full-body kissing, and learned to find your man's X-spots, all in preparation for performing oral sex. But all this prefellatio fuss begs the question: What is it with men and blow jobs?

 Oral sex is a man's number-one fantasy. A *lack* of oral sex is a man's number-one complaint.

It seems that among men there is no greater fear than that of being handed a fellatio-free life sentence. Surveys have shown that the number-one male fantasy is oral sex (number two is having a threesome, in case you were wondering). Similarly, a lack of oral sex is often cited as a man's number one complaint in the bedroom. It's obvious, then, that men like receiving oral. But are blow jobs *really* that important to their overall sexual enjoyment? What drives the apparent obsession that some men seem to have with oral sex, and do we, as women, really need to satisfy it to satisfy them?

Oral Sex Goes Online

In vino veritas. It's Latin for "There is truth in wine." While alcohol may be the oldest truth serum, the Internet is a modern-day cocktail of anonymous camaraderie and anything-goes chat that can squeeze the truth out of even the most sober and tight-lipped among us. One need only join an online message-board discussion to see this phenomenon in electronic action. In fact, message boards offer one of the best, most brutally honest forums in which to ask men how they *really* feel about fellatio . . . or the lack thereof.

So, again in the line of duty, we picked a password and logged in. We posted a single, simple question regarding the importance of oral sex on a number of men's message boards. Our question was deliberately simple so that we could see where the question would naturally lead. Then we sat back, shared a bottle of vino, and watched the computer screen as the conversation took on a life of its own. What follows is the edited synopsis of the hundred or so messages we read before the wine kicked in. And yes, we made up the handles—anonymity on top of anonymity.

Our posted question: How important is fellatio to you?

2long: No more important than oxygen.

Mrrightnow: BJs should be a mandatory part of foreplay.

2long: Foreplay? I like it as the main course.

EastCoast1: LOVE oral but wifey not too keen.

Mrrightnow: Poor bastard. Try washing it better.

EastCoast1: Washed it so much I'm lucky it's still on.

Redhotone: My wife loves giving oral, loves receiving.

EastCoast1: What's her number?

2long: My GF does it, but my ex didn't. I missed it. Even got head from a hooker once.

Fetish123: Haven't had a hooker but have had a few threesomes, MMF, where F blows us both.

2long: !!! Wow.

Fetish123: Best one was when husband put a blindfold on his wife and she sucked us both, not knowing if she was sucking him or me.

EastCoast1: Husband was into it?

Fetish123: Totally into it. Watching a guy get pleasure from being blown is incredible.

2long: That's true. I like watching porn with a guy getting head while I'm getting it. Like to watch in the mirror while she sucks, too.

Fetish123: 2long, what was hooker experience like?

2long: Not great. Too freaked about cooties.

Fetish123: Were you able to go thru with it?

2long: Well, I did pay in advance...

EastCoast1: Thought about hiring hooker for BJ. Looked through the escorts in the yellow pages when wife was out of town but lost the nerve.

Redhotone: I've been married 12 years. Never had a hooker or a 3some. Whatever you crave in bed, find a way to get your wife to give it to you. Better and safer in the long run.

MadMan2007:   For me, BJs are a must. I'll return the favor, but if she won't go down I won't stick around. Feels way too good to deny.

Redhotone: You shouldn't have to "deny" yourself anything. I can't imagine a lifetime of no oral. It's a big part of our sex life.

Flavorpot: Hey EastCoast, tell her BJs prevent cancer. I read it in a joke medical article.

MadMan2007:   Ha, I remember that article. Sent it to my GF at the time, but she was a doctor. Maybe that's why she gave such good head, knowing male anatomy so well! Ooh how I miss her...

Flavorpot: Best BJs are from women who love to do it.

Fetish123:   So true. Love it when a woman loses herself in it...Love holding her hair back and watching her bob up and down in your lap.

Redhotone: My wife sometimes fingers my ass when she's doing it. That's good, too.

Fetish123:   Sucking on balls works for me. Love girls who don't forget the balls.

Flavorpot: They're the best.

Who knew girls that "don't forget the balls" were held in such high esteem? See what you can learn online? Ball recall aside, eavesdropping on this discussion reveals a truth: Oral sex is important to men, and they appreciate it when a woman performs it with eager enjoyment.

My husband loves oral and I like doing it, but sometimes the smell and taste turn me off. How can I tactfully handle this without hurting his feelings?

♀ *Debra:* Share a shower and go down on him. Tell him you love the taste and smell of him when he's so fresh and clean. If he loves oral, he'll connect the dots. Also, be aware that diet can affect the way semen tastes. Meat, dairy, alcohol, and strong seasonings like garlic are thought to worsen taste, while fruits and veggies are thought to improve it.

♂ *Don:* Guys often aren't as sensitive about these kinds of things as women are. You'd probably be mortified if he asked you to wash or if he said he got a hair stuck in the back of his throat, but lots of men wouldn't be so embarrassed. It's good to be lighthearted about sex whenever you can. It takes the edge off. Smile and tell him you "don't do dirty things," then run the shower. When he's in there, hand him a pair of grooming scissors or a razor and ask him to play Edward Scissorhands. Tell him you'll be waiting eagerly in bed to see the results. He'll be too excited to be embarrassed.

8 The Art of Fellatio

Fellatio is one of the most intimate, loving, pleasurable activities that a couple can experience. Yet despite the sexual culture all around us, fellatio is still often regarded as a dirty, subservient, and even degrading sexual act performed primarily by slutty women. It isn't rocket science to figure out that this negative social attitude toward the fellatrix is at least partly to blame for some women's hesitancy to engage in, or to fully enjoy, performing fellatio. If you're one of them, we sympathize: Vulgar slang for oral sex— phrases like *cock sucking*—doesn't make a woman feel like a lady. The word *blow job*, while not exactly pretty, is nonetheless prevalent and is used in *Lip Service* (to replace it with *fellatio* at every turn would sound prudishly awkward).

The attitude shown by some men toward both fellatio and the fellatrix doesn't help matters, either. Many women have heard guys speak derogatorily of a girl who "sucked them off," "blew them," or whose mouth/throat/face was the amazed recipient of his ample load/wad/funk, and so forth. The porn industry—although it is getting better with the growth of the couples market and the presence of female filmmakers—further perpetuates the myth that oral sex is a dirty thing. It's difficult to feel wholesome about performing fellatio when the open-mouthed starlet on the screen is being pushed from erection to erection like a human vacuum cleaner whose bag is full.

It is important, then, to separate the way popular culture and some pornography presents fellatio from the way you and your lover personally feel about it. The truth is, blow jobs can bring excitement, variety, mutual sexual pleasure, and emotional closeness into a couple's sex life. If you can tune out what others say about fellatio (or how they say it), you can "go down" with pride and passion.

A Rose by Any Other Name . . .

Brianne and Munroe are longtime lovers, both in their mid-thirties, who only recently introduced regular fellatio into their sex life.

"Brianne would do it off and on," says Munroe, "but she'd never finish. She'd suck halfheartedly for a minute or two and then do something else. I wished she'd do it more. I asked for it lots, but that was all I ever got."

"Munroe would say, 'Will you blow me tonight, hon?'" Brianne reveals. "I *hated* that expression. It sounded adolescent and made me feel cheap. It's not that I don't like dirty talk. I like it a lot, but the timing has to be right; otherwise it's just trashy."

Although a rose by any other name would smell as sweet, Brianne is not alone in her aversion to off-color slang for fellatio. Words can pack a powerful punch, and they can influence our emotions. It may seem strange, but a woman who says, "I want to suck your cock" in the heat of the moment, may still be turned off when asked to "suck my cock."

So how did this tongue-tied couple finally resolve their verbal woes?

"I broke down and told Munroe how much I hated the way he asked for oral sex," says Brianne. "He had no idea how much it bothered me and asked how he could request it more respectfully. I gave him a few ideas. I didn't want him to verbally ask for it. I preferred that he gently direct my head toward his groin. If I didn't want to do it, I'd just shake my head."

"She doesn't shake her head very much," says a now-satisfied Munroe.

The point of Brianne and Munroe's story isn't to examine diction. The point is to encourage you to reflect upon *anything* that may be preventing you from performing the best fellatio possible, from terminology and past experience to your partner's attitude and the smell of his genitals, and to solve the problem as a couple. If you can, there will be no reason to omit this delightful but undeservedly defamed act from your sex life.

The "Top 10" Blow-Job Basics

Before we get into the specifics of oral sex, let's cover ten blow-job basics:

- Think of your own comfort when choosing a position. For example, place a towel under your knees if you're kneeling on the bathroom floor.

- Breathe through your nose and focus on keeping your jaw muscles relaxed.
- Incorporate hand strokes into fellatio to avoid mouth/jaw fatigue. (Several hand-job moves are described under "Helping Hands," below.)
- Use sufficient lubrication—that is, keep your mouth moist and use lots of saliva. Place a glass of water nearby to wet your whistle now and then.
- Cover your teeth with your lips and don't bite or scrape his genitals.
- Don't make a scene if you get a hair in your mouth. Keep stroking him with one hand while you discreetly fish it out with the other.
- Find pleasure in your performance. Watch how aroused your man is and let his arousal stir yours. If the position of your bodies allows, you can ask him to finger your genitals or pinch your nipples while you fellate him.
- Practice safe sex. If you're a long-term, healthy monogamous couple, this may simply entail cleanliness, and a barrier if analingus is part of your sex play. If you're new to each other or not monogamous, this may mean using a condom.
- Use what you have learned in *Lip Service*—everything from dirty talk and setting the mood to full-body kissing and skin-tingling teasers—to prep him for fellatio.
- Remember that your mouth is a sexual organ, and always use it with skillful enthusiasm when performing fellatio. Don't let your ministrations deteriorate into a string of mindless head bobs in your man's lap.

The Three Ss: Sweet, Sinful, and Sultry

Remember the three styles of full-body kisses? The same trio of styles—sweet, sinful, and sultry—are equally appropriate in the performance of fellatio. (It may be worthwhile to flip back and

I love to give oral, and I think I'm pretty good at it. Maybe too good. My boyfriend comes WAY too soon during oral. That kind of ruins things for me, since he's limp right away and loses interest. Any advice?

♀ *Debra*: Is he inexperienced or just inconsiderate? If he's inexperienced, ask him to masturbate a few hours before you and he have (oral) sex. And maybe stick to hand jobs or inter-course until he's acquired some staying power, since oral sex is intensely orgasmic for most men. If he is experienced, maybe he just needs to consider your pleasure before his own. Remind him what "ladies first" means.

♂ *Don*: Let him have his turbo BJ sometimes. They're fantas-tic. Other times, tell him you want to delay gratification; it'll make for a much stronger orgasm. When you're delaying things, don't let him get any kind of climactic momentum going. Do lots of starting and stopping. Suck, then stop and kiss his lips. Suck, then stop and ask him to touch you. You get the idea.

review "The Three Ss" in chapter 4.) Each style of fellatio creates a unique erotic aura that will have a different effect on your man's libido, thereby leading to distinct oral-sex experiences.

Generally speaking, a sweet style of fellatio fosters a soothing, romantic, emotionally bonding form of arousal and pleasure; a sinful style ignites the raunchier, more aggressive side of the male sex drive, resulting in a "nastier" blow-job experience; a sultry style fuels a man's self-indulgent desire, leading to an exquisitely sensual, highly passionate fellatio encounter.

As you did with the full-body kiss, be sure to choose one style and stick to it for the entire blow job. Your choice will depend on several factors, including your man's sexual longings, his emotional mood, the erotic mood you've set as well as your location (Are you in the bedroom or the backseat?) and circumstances (Are the kids at home? Are you wearing leather or lace?).

Variety of style is another important consideration. If you've been with your partner for a long time and regularly engage in fellatio, you may not even realize how homogenous or... well... *boring* your blow jobs have become. Think about how you usually perform fellatio and then choose the style that least resembles your natural style. Is your default oral-sex setting stuck on sweet? If so, crank the dial, ditch the good-girl act, and surprise him with a sinful bad-girl blow job.

As we've said, it's best to maintain one consistent style throughout a full-body kiss. The same holds true for fellatio. It is possible, however, to effectively switch styles *between* the body kiss and fellatio. For example, you can follow a sultry body kiss with a sinful blow job. A sweet body kiss followed by a sultry blow job is another nice combination. That being said, you should stay within one style until you have mastered both arts. There's no need to rush; you have a lifetime to experiment with combos.

Fellatio and the Fantasy Factor

When choosing the style of fellatio you want to perform, keep in mind any male fantasy elements that may be engaged by the body kiss, and be sure to keep them alive as you move into oral sex. If you're working against a deadline and have skipped the full-body foreplay, immersing your man in a fantasy is a quick and easy way to achieve the style of fellatio you want to perform.

Do you and your man want the blow job done with sultry decadence? Handcuff him to the headboard and show off your oral skills by fulfilling The Power Struggle fantasy on his penis. Would you prefer to do the job with even more haste and heat? Push him Up Against a Wall, drop to your sinful knees, and swallow his hard-on with all the desperate desire your mouth can muster. If you have a sweet tooth, bite into the Blow Jobs for Beginners role play to let your innocent, inexperienced tongue lick its way up and down his length, exploring and discovering every inch of him.

To exploit the common male fantasy of multiple partners within an oral-sex context and to use all three styles of fellatio in one encounter, consider using the following additional fantasy:

The Fivesome

This role play improves upon the standard threesome fantasy by bringing even more excitement—and two more make-believe mouths—into the mix as your man is lip-serviced by a grand total of four eager women. It goes something like this: You are a skilled fellatrix, and your advice is regularly sought by your friends, all of whom are constantly asking for tips and techniques to better fellate their boyfriends. To help your friends, and to give your man a night of unparalleled pleasure, you ask three of your friends to join you and your lucky partner for a night of practical instruction.

Have your man lie on his back on the bed. Either blindfold him or ask him to close his eyes. Tell him to imagine there are four women kneeling on the bed beside his body. You are between his legs. You begin to fellate him, demonstrating the sweet style of fellatio to your friends. A few moments later, a different mouth wraps around his cock to practice the sweet style. Next, you demonstrate the sultry style for a while before letting your second friend practice. Last, you demonstrate the sinful style, and your remaining friend slips in to practice, bringing your man to a wild and wonderful climax.

As you work your way through this fellatio fantasy, be sure to pause between make-believe mouths. This lets your man imagine that you and your friends are taking turns on him. To heighten this imaginary effect, focus on performing each style as distinctly as possible.

The Fivesome is an indulgent, raunchy role play that will quickly and completely captivate your man's imagination. It will skyrocket his arousal, whether or not you have first performed a full-body kiss. Perhaps most important, this particular fantasy facilitates the use of all three fellatio styles in one oral-sex session. For your man, this means receiving an onslaught of incredibly intense yet very distinct sensations. The effect is mind and body blowing.

Kiss Classification

Genital kissing is a fundamental part of fellatio. The types of kisses you use on your man's genitals therefore play a big part in his pleasure. With only minor modifications, the types of kisses you used during body kissing (in chapter 4) can also be used during genital kissing. For example:

The French kiss: This deep, open-mouthed tongue kiss feels great when performed on and under your man's scrotum and particularly on the perineum. Pretend this sensitive spot is his mouth and kiss it with the same passion.

The nibble: While as a rule you should keep your teeth clear of your partner's sensitive genitals, some men do enjoy gentle nibbles and teeth action once they are aroused. The glans and the shaft can respond well to soft love bites. Grazing the coronal ridge with your teeth is another pleasure possibility.

The suck: The suck's role in fellatio is obvious. Varying degrees of suction on the glans and shaft is an integral part of a blow job. How much of your man's shaft you take into your mouth to suck is also relevant. Tenderly sucking your man's testicles—a practice called tea bagging—is another form of sucking enjoyed by many men.

The tongue swirl: This is an essential kiss for good fellatio. Swirling your tongue around your man's aroused, swollen glans and along the smooth skin of his erect shaft feels exquisite. You can add variety to the tongue swirl by using just the tip of your tongue or by sticking your tongue out further and using the entire thick, fleshy organ. Tongue swirls also feel different when your lips are wrapped around his glans or shaft rather than when just your tongue makes contact with his skin.

The lick: The lick has nearly unlimited potential during oral sex. It is capable of great variety (from short and hard to long and luxurious) and can be used anywhere on his genitals.

The butterfly: For an ever-so-subtle sensation, flutter your eyelashes over your partner's glans. This is best done when his arousal is just mounting, as it may not be enough stimulation after he's felt more intense contact.

The hot tamale: Exhale hot breath onto your man's glans, erect shaft, scrotum, and/or perineum. These areas are highly receptive to stimulation.

The cool front: Immediately after performing the hot tamale, pull your head back and lower the temperature by exhaling cool air onto his glans, erect shaft, scrotum, and/or perineum. If he shudders, it's from pleasure, not the cold!

The Eskimo kiss: Nuzzle your nose into your partner's pubic hair. This lets you stimulate this often neglected area while keeping your mouth clear of hair.

The rimmer: In addition to analingus, rimming the coronal ridge is a guaranteed feel-good move. It's particularly pleasant as your tongue glides over the area of the ultrasensitive frenulum.

The flicker: A quick flick with the tip of your tongue can spike your man's arousal fast and hard. Tease his glans, coronal ridge, shaft, scrotum, perineum, and/or anus with a well-timed, well-placed tongue flick to send an unexpected rush of sensation to his groin.

The Three Ps: Pace, Pattern, and Pressure

Like a full-body kiss, the physical performance of fellatio is affected by the three variables of pace, pattern, and pressure. (Again, we recommend that you take a quick look back at "The Three Ps" in chapter 4 to reacquaint yourself with their different qualities.) The three Ps work together to let you perform the style of fellatio you desire, be it sweet, sinful, or sultry.

The pace of a blow job is the speed at which it is performed and, usually, how long it lasts. Speaking generally, a slow-paced blow job will last the longest and is therefore best for the sultry style, while a medium pace suits a medium-length sweet style. A fast pace supports the desperate erotic energy of the sinful style

I don't really know my boyfriend's history. He wears a condom during intercourse, but he's asking for a BJ without it because he says it feels better. Does it really make that much difference? Can I catch anything from oral sex?

♂ *Don:* To answer you with brutal honesty, wearing a condom is like eating a good meal with a numb tongue. But so what? This is your life. If this is going to be a lasting, exclusive relationship—and only if—both of you need to get tested for everything under the sun before you let him take the rubber off.

♀ *Debra:* You can catch any number of nasties during unprotected oral sex: everything from HIV to herpes. Visit a sexual health clinic or a reputable online sex health column before you even step into the same room as your boyfriend again. You need some sexual education, and you need it now. Your health is infinitely more important than a boyfriend's pleasure.

and will help you carry out a frantic fellatio quickie at breakneck speeds—he won't know what hit him!

A fellatio pattern is the path your genital kisses will follow. It may be regular and predictable (for example, starting at the glans and proceeding to the base, then repeating), or it may be unpredictable (perhaps beginning at the perineum, moving to the anus, and then jumping to the frenulum). Yet regardless of how your mouth travels over your man's genitals, its itinerary should be planned in advance to ensure a natural, uninterrupted flow. A good pattern can help your man's desire build at a steadily pleasurable rate. A poor or helter-skelter pattern can distract him and detract from his pleasure.

Pressure is the amount of force you use when performing oral sex. Like pace and pattern, the amount of pressure you use to lick, kiss, suck, and stroke your partner's genitals will assist you in carrying out the different styles of fellatio. Gentle "experimental" kisses suggest a sweetly innocent style. Confident, firm pressure is perfect for the sultry style. A hard, eager, almost painful level of pressure will help create a sinful style of fellatio and bring an exciting new edge to his experience. Varying the amount of pressure you use to deliver any type of kiss, from a lick to a rimmer, can also increase the kissing types at your disposal. For example, a soft suck and a hard suck—although classified the same—are nonetheless two very different types of kisses.

Practicing the three Ps of pace, pattern, and pressure is vital when learning to master the art of oral sex. When you learn to use the three Ps together, and to exploit the endless pleasure possibilities

Remember the one, two, threes of a body kiss? They're the same for fellatio:

- Choose a style: sweet, sinful, or sultry.
- Use a variety of kissing types, from the French to the flicker.
- Establish a flow through pace, pattern, and pressure.

they can create, you can provide your partner with an almost unlimited variety of both sexual sensations and oral-sex encounters.

Fellatio Positions

The position your man's body is in while receiving fellatio can have a significant impact on the sensations he experiences. One reason is novelty: Receiving oral sex in new or different positions can add fresh excitement to fellatio sessions that may have become stale. This is especially the case with long-term couples. The second reason is the differing angles of the penis. The exact same stroke can elicit completely different sensations, depending on the position of your man's body and the consequent angle of his erection. Even a minor shift—say, spreading his legs wider or bending his knees—can change the way your mouth feels.

Here are a few positions you may want to try.

HIM STANDING, HER KNEELING The standing position offers your man a terrific view not only of your naked body but also of his own erection as it disappears into your mouth. How delicious! This position also lets you grip his hips and buttocks, urging him to thrust deeper into your mouth. Your position—on your knees—lets him feel somewhat dominant and indulges his sexual ego, particularly if you let him hold on to your head to direct you.

HIM STANDING, HER LYING Have your man stand beside the bed while you lie on your back, your head hanging over the edge. Grip his penis from below, and then gently bend it downward so that you can take it in your mouth. Your man can lean over your body to rest his hands on the bed for support as you suck him from underneath. This position gives him a great view of your naked body below him. Because you're mostly immobile, your partner will have to do the thrusting in this position. Take it slow, and make sure he doesn't get too rammy until you're accustomed to this position; after all, this is an exciting arrangement.

♥ Some men love to play an active role in fellatio and revel in the freedom of being able to pump at will, especially as fellatio is often a passive, "hold-still" experience for men. The man-above position, as well as a couple of the others suggested here, facilitate a *sense* of domination and subservience that may arouse your man; however, always be sure that you are in *actual* control when performing fellatio. Unless your sexual trust is rock solid and you are confident in his ability to restrain himself, stick to positions where you are calling the shots. Fellatio is something you should enjoy as well, and you won't if you're worried about your gag reflex.

HIM SITTING, HER KNEELING Whether he's reclining in his favorite chair or perched on the edge of the bed, this is a classic position for a man to receive lip service. He can sit back and relax as your warm mouth works its wonders between his open legs. If he's sitting on the floor or the edge of the bed, have him lean back on his arms / elbows, and spread his legs wider than usual for a little variety.

HIM STRADDLING HER CHEST Ask your man to straddle your chest, facing you. Grip his erection and guide it toward your mouth, encouraging him to thrust into it. If you wish, you can wrap your arms around him to grip and knead his buttocks, thereby leaving the force and rhythm of his thrusts up to him.

SIXTY-NINE There are a few sixty-nine positions you may want to try: (1) Sit on his chest, facing his feet, and lean over to suck him. Your bum and genitals will be close to his face, thus giving him the opportunity to gaze at your goods or even lick/finger you. Many men are turned on by an aroused woman, so let yourself feel pleasure, and you'll naturally increase his. (2) Both you and he can lie on your sides, facing different directions. (3) He can kneel above you on all fours, facing your feet, so that you suck him from underneath. This position can bend his erection back quite a bit, which can be pleasurable, but proceed with caution until you know his comfort limits.

HIM LYING ON HIS BACK An advantage of the horizontal position is that your man can completely relax his body and lose himself in the experience. It's also a comfortable position for you, too, since you can recline alongside his body. If you lie with your head toward his, he can reach down and hold your head—or at least clutch your hair—when the mood strikes. If you lie with your head toward his feet, he can finger you as you work on him. Crouching or lying on your stomach between his legs is another user-friendly position for you to assume. To jazz up this standard-issue position, have your man hook his elbows behind his knees to hold his legs up and apart as you service him. This fosters an enticing sense of exposure and vulnerability.

HIM ON HIS KNEES Have your man kneel on the bed or floor, and lie on your belly in front of him. If your mouth can't comfortably reach his genitals, ask him to lower his body or rest on his haunches and spread his knees so you can get the access you need.

HIM ON ALL FOURS With your man on all fours, snake underneath him—your head in the same direction as his—so that your face is under his genitals. Ask him to push his erection past your lips and to pump. Since you can use your forearms to push up against his body, thereby indicating if he's thrusting too hard or deep, this position is a good one to use if you want to let him play boss.

When it comes to body positions for fellatio, the position of *your* body is also something to consider as it, too, can bring variety to your partner's experience. Think of a man who normally receives oral sex while lying on his back, his woman between his legs, his usual view being the top of her head: If she shakes things up by jumping on top of him and doing a one-eighty (thus getting into the sixty-nine position), he can now enjoy the rousing sight of her bum and genitals as she sucks him. It's a nice change, isn't it? Remember that great oral sex is as much about variety and excitement as it is about technique. Keep fellatio fresh, and you'll avoid a stale sex life.

Hand-to-Mouth

While it's possible to perform a totally hands-free blow job, most are made much better when you get your hands a little dirty. Incorporating basic hand-job moves into oral sex not only increases your

My boyfriend is a great lover. The problem is, he can last too long during oral sex. I think I'm getting TMJ. Do you have any magic tricks that'll make him come on demand?

♂ *Don:* Does he last a long time because he has good endurance or because he's distracted by something? Does he seem frustrated by how long it takes him? Guys get distracted, too. Before you assume this is a bedroom issue, talk to him and see if anything is bothering him. Oh, yeah, and don't forget to play with his balls. We like that.

♀ *Debra:* A sudden shift in momentum can often help a guy reach orgasm. If you're stroking slowly, switch to a fast stroke. Touch yourself and tell him you can't wait to taste him. Tossing in a different technique, such as an unexpected twist to the glans, can also help him get there. That's providing he *wants* to get there. If he's prolonging oral sex on purpose, tell him your jaw is tiring (you're only human!) and you may have to switch to using your hands. If he wants to come in your mouth, he'll pick up the pace.

partner's pleasure by varying the sensations he feels but it also ensures that your mouth and jaw don't become fatigued.

Since you'll need a lot of lubrication for your hand strokes, be sure to coat his erection with your saliva before using your hands. (Unless you have a flavored favorite, you may not want to use an artificial lube during oral sex.) During fellatio, do a series of moist mouth strokes, then smoothly transition into two or three manual strokes before again using your mouth. Both of your hands should be busy: one holding or stroking the shaft, the other stimulating the scrotum. Some must-have manual moves include:

The ring: Make a ring with your index finger and thumb and encircle the base of your partner's penis to hold it steady while you perform fellatio. If you squeeze tightly, your index finger and thumb can act as a natural cock ring. Sliding the ring up and down is a simple but very stimulating hand stroke that can accompany your mouth strokes.

The fingertip stroke: Starting at the base of his penis, drag your fingertips up his shaft and then back down.

The fire starter: Place his erect penis between your palms and roll your hands back and forth, rubbing it as though trying to start a fire.

Twist the lid: To add an unexpected twist to almost any hand stroke, twist the head of his penis as the stroke ends.

Heavenly hands stroke: Place his penis between your hands, with your fingers pointing upward, as if you're praying. Press your hands together tightly, and slide them up and off his erection.

The palm press: Place the palm of one hand directly on top of the glans and press down.

The leveler: Put your hands close together and slide both palms over the underside of his penis, starting at the base and moving up, thus pressing his erection flat against his belly. You can start this stroke under the scrotum as well; just push it upward, and let your palms glide over it en route to his erection.

Finger-laced stroke: Lace your fingers together and stroke his shaft with your palms. This stroke is great because it lets you deliver high-pressure strokes without cramping your hands. It also makes your partner's penis feel snugly enclosed.

The milkmaid stroke: This is an upward-only stroke. Picture milking a cow, and imagine that you're milking his erection the same way by repeatedly pulling your tight grip from the base to the glans.

The squeeze: Wrap your fingers around his erect shaft and squeeze rhythmically, giving him pulses of pressure and pleasure.

The claw: Curl your fingers under to resemble claws and hook your fingertips under the coronal ridge. Squeeze the glans as you pull your fingertips up and over the ridge.

The ball bounce and tug: Bounce your partner's testicles in your hand and then oh-so-tenderly pull on them. You can pull on his pubic hair, too.

The perineum press: Press your fingers, thumb, or knuckles against his perineum as you suck or stroke him.

The wrist twist: Wrap your hand around his erection, with your pinkie down. Squeeze and stroke down to the base. Pull your fist up and off his erection, quickly twisting your wrist, so that your thumb is down. Squeeze and stroke down to the base. Pull your fist back upward, again twisting your wrist into the pinkie-down position for the next downstroke. The wrist twist is a good move because it facilitates fast stroking. The contrasting wrist positions also make your fist feel different with each and every stroke, since your thumb can squeeze tighter than your pinkie.

The penetrator II: Because your tongue can't be in two places at once (too bad!), you can instead penetrate your partner's anus with a finger during fellatio. The prostate, sometimes referred to as the male G-spot, can be reached by inserting a finger a few inches into the rectum, and curling it upward to stroke him internally (think of the "come here" finger curl). The deeply pleasurable sensation that results can lead to strikingly powerful orgasms, especially when combined with fellatio.

Unless it's a real mouth marathon, you won't use all of these hand manipulations during an oral-sex session. Alternate the strokes and combinations of strokes you use, and you'll have an almost endless supply of hand-to-mouth techniques with which to skillfully service your man.

As always, remember the importance of both the fellatio style you've chosen and the role of the three Ps. Should you tease his shaft with a light, feathery fingertip stroke, or torment it with a firm, raking fingertip stroke? Should your strokes be nice or nasty? It

Hand strokes at a glance:

- The ring
- The fingertip stroke
- The fire starter
- Twist-the-lid
- The heavenly hands stroke
- The palm press
- The leveler
- The finger-laced stroke
- The milkmaid stroke
- The squeeze
- The claw
- The ball-bounce-and-tug
- The perineum press
- The wrist twist
- The penetrator II

depends on whether you're working in the sweet or sinful style. Make sure your hands follow your lips' lead, and you can't go wrong.

Blow-Job Blueprints

The "blow-job blueprint" is the final product of all your study and skill. It is where everything you've learned about the art of fellatio comes together, enabling you to plan and perform the ultimate oral-sex experience. Similar to the body blueprints outlined in chapter 4, blow-job blueprints are essentially mental flowcharts that you'll keep in mind as you perform fellatio. Each blow-job blueprint incorporates the style of fellatio you've chosen; the types of kisses you'll use; the pace, pattern, and pressure with which you'll proceed; and the hand strokes you'll include.

While these blow-job blueprints are of obvious value to the novice fellatrix, they're also useful to the veteran whose sucks and strokes have become unimaginative or uninspired. In a long-term relationship, it's all too easy to fall back on the safety of the same old sex moves. Yet even if a woman has been performing fellatio for many years, these blueprints will help her think outside the blow-job box. Ultimately, a blueprint's value stems not from any secret technique or order but from its ability to motivate a woman to perform fellatio with creativity, enthusiasm, variety, affection, and skill. And once a woman can do that, she can draw up her own master blueprint.

BLOW-JOB BLUEPRINT A

Position of partner: Sitting
Style: Sweet
Pace: Medium
Pattern: Repeating, glans to base
Pressure: Partner's usual preference
Types of kisses used: Eskimo, butterfly, lick, suck, tongue swirl
Hand strokes: The ring, fingertip stroke, the squeeze, fire
  starter, the milkmaid

Regardless of whether you've primed your man with a partial- or full-body kiss, it's time to treat him to an edge-of-his-seat oral delight. Once he's unclothed, have him scoot to the edge of the bed and lean back on his hands to make his genitals accessible to you. For a change of scenery, serve this sweet treat in the kitchen or living room: Ask him to sit back in his chair or on the couch while you kneel between his legs. It's best if you're completely naked so that he can look down to admire your breasts, perhaps reaching down to touch them as his arousal builds.

Push your partner's legs wide apart, and, keeping your hands at your sides and your lips closed, nuzzle your nose into his pubic hair for an erotic Eskimo kiss. As he begins to harden, hold his shaft gently in your hand and place several butterfly kisses on the head of his penis. Next, position your fingertips at the base of his penis and slide them up and down the smooth skin of his shaft, covering the sides as well as the upper and undersides. If he's still flying at half-mast, the feeling of these fingertip strokes should send his erection skyward.

Wrap your index finger and thumb around the base of his erect shaft to form a ring. Using the ring to hold his erection steady, lick the glans with just the tip of your tongue before flattening your tongue (this will cover more surface area) and licking the glans like the top of an ice cream cone. Still holding his erection in place with the ring, purse your lips and place them against the glans as if you're going to take him in your mouth, but wait. Make the most out of this agonizingly anticipatory moment by looking up and making eye contact with your man.

If you're playing the part of the nervous first-time fellatrix, press the glans of his penis against your tight lips as though hesitating to let it penetrate your mouth. This creates a resistance on the head of his penis that stretches back the skin and feels excruciatingly good. Wait for the telltale thrust of his hips to betray his agony before letting his glans squeeze through your pursed lips. Slide your mouth down, then back up his shaft. Perform a tongue swirl on the glans before pulling your mouth off his erection.

To let your partner soak up this initial storm of sensation, wrap your hand around his shaft and simply squeeze it in rhythmic pulses. Again form the ring around the base of his penis and push your mouth onto his erection, going down as far as you can. Maintain this position and stick out your tongue to lick around his shaft. Slide your mouth up and down his shaft, coating it with saliva for good lubrication.

To stave off jaw fatigue, take breaks from your mouth maneuvers to fall back on a few hand moves. The fire-starter stroke will keep him hot while you rest: Place his penis between your hands and rub briskly. Take him in your mouth again, stroking up and down. Remember that you can combine a sliding ring stroke with your mouth to give him the sensation that his entire length is going into your mouth.

Mouth-stroke him until you tire, and then switch to a milkmaid stroke for variety: One hand should hold a ring at the base of his shaft to keep it steady and act as a cock ring, while the other hand strokes upward in a milking motion. Repeat several times before again pushing his glans past your lips. Slide your mouth down his shaft. Look up and keep eye contact while you fellate him. Maintain this hand-to-mouth routine until he reaches orgasm.

Blow-Job Blueprint A at a glance:

- Have your man sit as you kneel between his open legs.
- Nuzzle your nose in his pubic hair to help him harden.
- Place butterfly kisses on the glans, and stroke his shaft with your fingertips.
- Form a ring to hold his shaft at the base, and then lick the glans.
- After some resistance, let his erection push past your lips.
- Mouth-stroke his erection, and lick his shaft.
- Perform a few fire-starter and sliding-ring hand strokes.
- Alternate your mouth strokes with milkmaid hand strokes until he comes.

BLOW-JOB BLUEPRINT B

Position of partner: Supine
Style: Sultry
Pace: Slow
Pattern: Repeating, anus to glans
Pressure: Light, average, and strong
Types of kisses used: French, flicker, lick, suck, rimmer, tongue swirl, hot tamale, cool front, nibble

Hand strokes: The ring, heavenly hands, the wrist twist, twist-the-lid, the leveler, the perineum press, penetrator II

Blow-Job Blueprint B is a sexual endurance test for you and your man. How long can you fellate? How long can he withhold his orgasm? This sensorial masterpiece of the mouth will push both of you to your limits. But exhaustion has never been so enjoyable.

Your man should be lying naked on his back, his knees bent and his legs spread apart. You should be between his legs, either kneeling or lying on your stomach. To begin, lift his scrotum and gently French-kiss his perineum. Holding his scrotum out of the way, gently touch his anus with the index finger of your other hand, and at the same time increase the intensity of the perineal French kiss. Don't penetrate his anus with your finger, but simply apply pressure to it.

While maintaining light pressure on his anus, begin to flick your tongue over his scrotum. Lick around its perimeter. As his arousal mounts, suck on his testicles in turn, drawing each into your mouth (tea-bagging) with as much force as he likes. When he is fully erect, deliver a long lick to the underside of his shaft, extending all the way from the base to the frenulum. Form a ring around the base of his penis and bring his glans to your mouth. Beginning at the frenulum, use just the tip of your tongue to rim around the coronal ridge.

Apply slightly more pressure to his anus. Give him another long lick from the base of his penis to the frenulum, topping it off with another rimmer around the coronal ridge. Repeat this a few times before taking just the glans in your mouth and performing several tongue swirls on it. Return your attention to his perineum: Restimulate this area with a tongue swirl, followed by a hot-tamale and cool-front combo. Lick and suck his testicles again, carrying one of the licks up the underside of his penis to the glans.

Push your lips past the glans and swallow as much of his shaft as you can. Perform a few basic up-and-down mouth strokes, with or without a sliding ring stroke, to lubricate his erection. Hold it steady with a ring at the base. Nibble very gently along the sides and underside of the shaft. Return to the basic mouth stroke, gradually increasing your suction from mild to strong. Make sure to increase the finger pressure on his anus as your sucks get stronger.

Take a breather and place your heavenly hands in the prayer position, with one hand on either side of his shaft. Squeeze and slide your hands up and down his erection. Repeat as many times as you like. If you need more lubrication, interrupt your prayers for a few mouth strokes. For variety, switch hand strokes and perform several wrist twists, topping off every third one with a twist-the-lid to the glans.

Return to mouth strokes. At this point, your suction should be fairly strong, as should the pressure of the finger ring around his shaft. Starting at the perineum, perform a string of leveling strokes: Roll his scrotum up along the underside of his shaft and keep sliding your palms upward, pushing his erection flat against his belly. Interrupt this string of hand strokes with lubricating mouth strokes. Vary the depth of each, sometimes swallowing his entire shaft, other times just the head. Deep-throat if you can. Tossing in an occasional twist-the-lid will add unexpected flares of sensation to his glans.

Because this blueprint involves anal penetration with a finger, you'll want to have some good artificial lubricant nearby. Use a thicker lube, preferably one designed for anal play. Coat your finger, ask your man to spread his legs wider, and *gently, slowly*

Blow-Job Blueprint B at a glance:

- Have your man lie on his back, with his knees bent and his legs apart.
- Lift his scrotum, and French-kiss his perineum while touching his anus.
- Lick and tongue-flick his scrotum, and gently suck on his testicles.
- Lick the underside of his shaft and rim the coronal ridge.
- Restimulate his perineum with kisses, and lick his testicles.
- Mouth-stroke his shaft, with or without a sliding-ring hand stroke.
- Increase the strength of your suction while applying more pressure to the anus.
- Perform several heavenly-hands strokes, and then return to mouth strokes.
- Perform several leveling hand strokes, interrupted by mouth strokes.
- Using lots of lube, penetrate his anus with a finger.
- Fellate him and stimulate his prostate until he climaxes.

penetrate his anus with your index finger. Twist your wrist so that your palm is facing upward and make the "come here" finger curl to stimulate his prostate. Keep the channels of communication open by asking him how it feels.

Return to fellatio—nothing fancy, just up-and-down mouth strokes—as you continue to stimulate him internally. Hum to show him how aroused you are and to create a slight vibration along his shaft. Continue in this way until he climaxes.

Blow-Job Blueprint C

Position of partner: Standing
Style: Sinful
Pace: Fast
Pattern: Repeating, glans to base
Pressure: Strong
Types of kisses used: Suck, nibble, lick, flicker
Hand strokes: The ring, finger-laced stroke, the claw, the palm
   press, ball bounce and tug

Compared with the skilled, sultry sexual excess of the previous blueprint, this one is a desperate, decadent quickie. Since it's a fast and nasty encounter, you may not always want to precede it with the luxury of a body kiss. That's okay; your man won't mind if you skip the preview and go straight to the main feature.

Because this is a somewhat sinful rendezvous, why not initiate contact while your man is still dressed? Push him against the wall, drop to your knees, and grope his groin with shameless passion. Bite through his clothing until you feel the telltale bulge of arousal, and then unzip his pants, pushing them down just enough to get to his genitals. Squeeze and nibble his bulge through his underwear and then push them down, too.

Hold his erection with a finger ring at the base. Dive onto his hardness with your mouth in one fast, strong mouth stroke. Use your mouth like a vacuum and pull it off his penis with good suction. Suck hard on the head as your mouth reaches the tip. If he enjoys it, you can gently graze the coronal ridge with your teeth as your mouth comes off. You can also nibble his glans and shaft. Some men are more sensitive than others when it comes to teeth, so take your cues from him.

Suck him again and continue as long as you like before gasping for breath and breaking with a finger-laced stroke. Lick and tongue-flick the glans and frenulum while holding his erection steady at the base with a ring. Return to sucking. Stop, form a claw with your fingers, and pull up on the coronal ridge. Pull upward until your fingertips slide over the glans, pinching it as they come off his penis. Follow this move with a firm palm press to the glans. This alternating claw–palm press combo nicely stimulates the head by first stretching and then compressing the skin.

Suck strongly, as though suddenly trying to bring him to a quick orgasm. One hand should be stabilizing his erection; the other hand should be clutching a hip or buttock, pulling his groin closer, and encouraging him to thrust harder. For added sensation, scrape the glans against your hard palate as you suck. Next, direct the angle of his erection toward the inside of your cheek, so that your cheek bulges with each of his thrusts. Make sure he watches; it's an unforgettable sight.

Scrotal stimulation is a big part of fellatio, and the standing position facilitates a very pleasurable ball-bounce-and-tug action. Hold his testicles in one hand and squeeze gently. Bounce them in your hand before tenderly tugging them away from his body. This will feel particularly good if you continue to fellate him while you squeeze, bounce, and pull.

Because this is a bad-girl blueprint, you may want to re-create a

Blow-Job Blueprint C at a glance:

- While standing, push your man against a wall and fondle his groin.
- Pull down his pants to stimulate his bulge through his underwear.
- Pull down his underwear and mouth-stroke him, sucking hard as you pull.
- Mouth-stroke him, interrupting fellatio with finger-laced hand strokes.
- Hold his erection with a ring at the base, and perform an alternating claw–palm press combo to the glans.
- Suck hard, letting him see your cheek bulge from his erection.
- Continue to fellate him while bouncing and tugging his testicles.
- Slap the underside of his glans against your flattened tongue.
- Fellate and hand-stroke him to orgasm.

few porn staples. First, grip your man's erection at the base: Open your mouth and stick out your flattened tongue, then repeatedly slap the underside of his glans against it. Make sure to keep eye contact. The visual of this move is as effective as the feel. Another technique often seen in porn involves a film fellatrix (or fellatrixes) dropping gobs or strings of saliva onto a man's erection before sucking it. Sure, this is great for lubrication, but your guy may not like the sight. Ask him what he thinks of this beforehand to avoid turning him off. Similarly, don't push yourself to do it if the idea or image is unappealing.

Continue to fellate and hand-stroke until your man reaches orgasm.

BLOW-JOB BLUEPRINT D

Position of partner: On all fours
Style: Sultry
Pace: Slow
Pattern: Repeating, base to glans
Pressure: Average and strong
Types of kisses used: Lick, suck, tongue swirl, flicker, hot tamale
Hand strokes: The ring, fire starter, ball-bounce-and-tug, perineum press, Penetrator II

This blueprint has you lying underneath your partner. Your heads should be pointing in the same direction, and your mouth should be directly underneath his genitals. As he crouches above you, ask him to lower his erection toward your lips. Form a finger ring around the base of his penis to hold it steady while you languidly lick the underside, base to frenulum. Suck the glans, and keep your lips around it as you smother it with slow tongue swirls.

Snake downward and/or ask him to lean forward so that you can kiss his perineum with alternating tongue swirls and flickers. Slowly move your mouth back up the underside of his shaft, warming this smooth, sensitive stretch of skin with a series of hot tamales. Bend his penis down toward your mouth to rapturously suck the glans before sliding your lips back down the shaft. Perform as many mouth strokes and sliding ring strokes as you like: You can

 Blow-Job Blueprint D at a glance:

- Have your man get onto all fours. Lie below him.
- Lick the underside of his shaft, and then kiss and suck the glans.
- Snake downward to kiss his perineum.
- Kiss the underside of his shaft.
- Bend his penis down so you can suck the glans and mouth-stroke the shaft.
- Alternate mouth strokes with sliding-ring and fire-starter strokes.
- Stimulate his perineum and testicles.
- Using lots of lube, penetrate his anus with a finger.
- Fellate and finger him until he comes.

alternate these with strong, slow fire-starter hand strokes, thus prolonging the experience and adding variety.

Passionately suck on his testicles. Bounce them in your hands and tug them away from his body. Press and massage his perineum. When you sense he's ready for anal play, lube your finger and reach behind his scrotum to finger his anus. Slowly slip your finger inside. Withdraw it just as slowly, repeating this as many times as he likes. Fellate and finger him simultaneously until he comes.

BLOW-JOB BLUEPRINT E

Position of partner: Sixty-nine
Style: Sinful
Pace: Fast
Pattern: Repeating, glans to base
Pressure: Strong
Types of kisses used: Lick, suck, tongue swirl, rimmer
Hand strokes: The ring, the squeeze

For a change of scenery, straddle your man's body so that you're facing his feet and he's gazing up at your genitals. Mount him with enthusiasm, and without further ado clutch the base of his penis with a finger ring while you lick and suck his glans. Swallow as much of his shaft as you can and bathe it with tongue swirls. Keep your lips tightly closed around his erection while you rim the coronal ridge with the tip of your tongue. With your lips still closed, slide the underside of your tongue over the glans.

Perform as many mouth strokes as you like, using as much suction as he can take. As always, you can accompany your mouth strokes with a sliding ring stroke to increase the pressure your man feels around his shaft and to impart a deep-throating sensation. When you need a break—or you want to delay his impending orgasm—stop sucking or stroking, and instead begin to rhythmically squeeze his shaft. Not that he'll need an invitation, but feel free to ask him to kiss or finger you while you fellate him. React with vocal pleasure when he does: Squirm and groan on top of him and suck/stroke with even more frantic desire. To really push him over the edge, encourage him to pump up into your mouth with powerful thrusts.

Don't be surprised if your man comes faster than usual during this blow job. This is a furiously passionate sixty-niner that ranks high on both the sensorial and visual scales. A little delayed gratification is okay, but don't make him wait too long. Sometimes short and sinful can be heavenly.

Blow-Job Blueprint E at a glance:

- Get into the sixty-nine position (woman on top).
- Kiss his glans, then swallow his shaft.
- With your lips around his erection, rim the coronal ridge with your tongue and lick the glans.
- Fellate him: To mimic deep throating, incorporate a sliding-ring stroke.
- Ask him to pump up into your mouth until he reaches orgasm.

Finish the Job

What's the point of sweating through a race, only to slow down as you approach the finish line? Orgasm and ejaculation may be the final products of fellatio, but there's no reason to relax as your man reaches them. His ultimate sexual release is an integral part of his fellatio experience. Technique, style, and variety still apply during climax. There are many ways you can maximize the eroticism of your man's orgasm and thus extend the pleasure of fellatio. Some of the possibilities are:

1. Keep your lips around his shaft and let him ejaculate in your mouth, maintaining eye contact as you swallow his come.
2. Keep your mouth wrapped around him, but let him watch as his come spills out.
3. Have him stroke himself and ejaculate into your waiting mouth.
4. Finish him off with hand strokes and let him ejaculate on your face or body.
5. Surprise him by assuming an inviting sexual position and begging him to come inside you.

9   Toys for Boys

A woman's mouth may be a powerful sexual organ, but that doesn't mean it has to function alone when performing oral sex. Male sex toys can ease its workload and exponentially increase a man's pleasure. Modern technology can make old-fashioned fellatio a thing of the past, so stock up on batteries and get ready to give him a buzz in the bedroom.

> Modern technology can make old-fashioned fellatio a thing of the past.

Press "On" for Pleasure

As we saw in chapter 3, certain passion props can be used to set an erotic mood for a full-body kiss and, ultimately, fellatio: Mirrors, music, pornography, even cybersex are all playthings that work on your man's mental arousal. While there is an element of mental arousal with sex toys—the novelty itself is exciting to many men—their primary purpose is to intensify physical pleasure.

In the same way that the erotic extras in chapter 5 (such as massage oils, fur, loofahs, whips, and hot-wax play) stimulate your man's skin to enhance his enjoyment of a full-body kiss, sex toys stimulate his genitals to heighten his pleasure during fellatio. The combination of your natural mouth and an artificial sex toy leads to amplified physical sensations and responses that neither your mouth nor the toy could achieve alone. By using both together, you do more than merely double his pleasure; you increase it multifold.

The combination of your mouth and a toy can amplify a man's sexual sensation.

A Pocketful of Pleasure

"Jae works out of town a lot," says his wife of six years, Sharon. "We're used to being apart in some ways. I handle the house, the finances, all that. But some things are harder to get used to. Like no sex. Unfortunately, Jae's absence means abstinence. It's impossible to get used to that part of it. It sucks."

"My line of work is a recipe for divorce," says Jae. "I see it all the time. Husbands have one-nighters on the road. Wives have affairs at home. It's cliché. I honestly don't think Sharon and I would ever fall into that trap, but we do joke about it. She'll say, 'Behave your-self,' when I leave, and I'll tell her to 'keep the doors locked,' when I go. We have phone sex now and then, too. That takes the edge off."

Wanting to do more than 'take the edge off' his wife's sexual longings, Jae presented her with a present on the eve of a long-term departure. It was a vibrator.

"I laughed when I opened it," says Sharon, "but I use it. *A lot.* In fact I was surprised how good it felt. I started to use it during our phone sex, and it made those orgasms stronger."

But fair's fair, isn't it? What about poor Jae's unsatisfied sexual needs?

"Sharon gave me a gift on the night before my next set away," recalls Jae. "I was expecting a couple of new books, so imagine my surprise when I opened it to find a pocket pussy. I didn't know what to make of it. I liked the idea of her using a vibrator, but I'd never used a pocket pussy before. I guess I'm old-fashioned. If I can't have the real thing, I just use my hand."

"He smiled but was obviously unsure about it," says Sharon. "I didn't know if he'd use it or not. It was a good toy—an artificial vagina that was supposedly a mold of some porn star. To me, a guy using that is no different than a woman using a vibrator."

Like they always did, Jae and Sharon spent the night before Jae's next long departure engaging in as much sexual activity as they could.

"I really wanted to make sure Jae would use the artificial vagina when he was away," Sharon continues, "so I decided to use it that night to show him how good it could feel."

"She'd been sucking me for a while," says Jae. "I could tell she was trying to make it last a long time, since she'd ease up every time I was close to coming. I was really worked up. She pulled the pocket pussy out of the nightstand and lubed it up while I watched. It turned me on to watch that. I started to wonder what it would feel like. She slid it onto my cock and *wow*, what a feeling. It felt tight and different. She started to fuck me with it, and my cock got totally engorged. And then, just when I thought it couldn't get any better, she started sucking on my balls. I think that was the best blow job I've ever had."

"The toy worked wonders," says Sharon. "It worked even better than I hoped it would. I kept pumping him with it while I licked his balls. His whole body went rigid, and he came really hard inside it. It was fantastic."

"And less hassle than another woman," jokes Jae.

Put Down Your Hand

Male masturbation toys are fantastically fun gifts to give your guy, and almost all will feel better than his hand. As with most sex toys, they come in a wide variety of styles, shapes, sizes, construction materials, and, of course, price ranges. Some are simple masturbation sleeves, with or without suction, while others are realistic replicas of a woman's mouth, vagina (like the porn-star pocket pussy Sharon gave Jae), or anus. Some vibrate to stimulate the glans, shaft, and/or testicles, while others come with a selection of differently textured openings and innards. All require the use of lube for effective stroking.

Regardless of the specific style you choose, a male masturbation toy can be used in various ways before or during fellatio. You

A male masturbation toy, from pocket pussies to penis pumps, can be used in various ways during fellatio.

can prep your man with it before using your mouth and thereby use it as foreplay. Or you can try it in lieu of hand strokes when your mouth gets tired and you need to take a break. These may not be the best options if you dislike the taste of lubricant, including flavored "blow-job" lubricant. If that's the case, use the toy to bring your man to climax as Sharon did: Pump his shaft with it, or have him hold it and thrust into it, while you stimulate his testicles or anus with your mouth.

The Ring of Fire

Penis rings are another pleasure possibility. Again, these come in a host of styles and are made of various materials, including rubber, latex, jelly, silicone, and Cyberskin. Penis rings wrap around the base of your man's shaft and work by trapping blood in the penis, thereby helping him maintain his erection longer. While some are simple utilitarian rings that look like they belong in the garage, others are colorful extraterrestrial-looking devices that boast ticklers (to stimulate a woman's vagina/clit/perineum/anus during intercourse) and vibrators (to stimulate both partners). If you prefer to go high tech, choose hands-free, wireless, ultra-quiet, and waterproof to get the most for your money.

Penis rings are the perfect choice if you're looking to treat your man to an extralong session of extrastrong oral sex. Slide one onto his penis and watch as his erection reaches new heights. You may even find that performing oral sex on him in the presence of the ring adds to your arousal.

Butt . . .

Sex toys can also add pleasure to anal play. Butt plugs, anal beads, vibrating probes, and dildos are available in all lengths and girths. Many are angled for ideal prostate massage, and—as if vibration weren't enough—some also inflate, rotate, and "ejaculate" water. If your heterosexual man is new to anal exploration, however, it's best to just use a well-lubed finger or perhaps a graduated string of anal beads, since these aren't as phallic as a probe or a plug.

Once again, be sure that the lube you choose is suitable for anal penetration. A thick water- or silicone-based lube is best, and there are many on the market. Always ask the salesperson for information or read the package of any and all sex products you purchase to ensure compatibility. For example, silicone lube is great for anal fingering, but it will break down silicone anal toys.

If your man is already accustomed to anal play, try introducing

Always make sure that your sex toys and your personal lubricants are compatible.

a remote-control butt plug into fellatio. Insert it into his anus and then ask him to sit on the edge of the bed with his legs spread. With the remote control in hand, begin to perform oral sex on him while stimulating his anus at your whim. The anticipation of the anal stimulation, and the feel of your mouth on his genitals, will result in the best blow job any man could imagine. Tack on a set of nipple clamps and he'll really squirm!

Get a Buzz

The vibrator is perhaps the classic sex toy. Although often thought of as a female sex toy, the vibrator can feel good to a man, too. For example, you can roll a straight or bullet/egg-type vibrator over your man's glans, shaft, and balls to give his genitals a deeply pleasurable tingle. Or, you can press the vibrator against his perineum and anus, experimenting with the different settings, perhaps even slipping it inside his anus. This type of sensation, particularly when combined with the feel of your hot, sucking mouth on his erection, is pure ecstasy. Fingertip vibrators are a sexy way to further refine your fine motor skills on his genitals.

A vibrating tongue is another fun option that may indulge your man's fantasies. These are often used to pleasure women, but there's

Vibrators aren't just for the fairer sex; they're great for guys, too.

no reason your man can't get in on the action. Once your man's erection is well lubed with your saliva, add the extra "tongue" and let him imagine he has two mouths working on him. You can suck him while the tongue teases his balls, perineum, and anus. It's the closest many men will ever get to a threesome!

Wrap It Up

While not as glamorous as these battery-powered feats of erotic engineering, the condom can also be a good sex toy, providing that you and your partner don't normally use them in your sex life. If you've been married or together for a long while, it may have been some time since your man felt a condom around his erection. If that's the case, slip one on him, and perform fellatio while he wears it. He can fall into a fantasy where he's single and getting a blow job from a stranger. Alternatively, you can suck him for a few minutes before removing it to once again let him fully appreciate the feel of your mouth on his cock.

10 : The Tailor-Made Blow Job

Even the highest-quality, most expensive designer suit needs to be tailored before it can hang perfectly on a man's shoulders. The same is true with oral sex. Even if a woman has learned to skillfully use her mouth as a sexual organ and has mastered the art of fellatio, she must still personalize her technique to satisfy her partner's unique preferences. This takes two things: practice and communication.

The truth is, many men who receive oral sex are just *so happy* to be experiencing fellatio, that they don't express their feel-good preferences for fear of offending the fellatrix. But if a job's worth doing, it's worth doing right. Right? Assuming you answered yes, we've included a handful of questions that you may wish to pose to your man in an effort to refine his oral pleasure.

If you and your partner have trouble speaking openly about your sexual desires, ask him to read these questions in private and to write down his answers. He can add new ideas whenever he wants, thereby using this book as a communication medium until you learn to speak more comfortably. If you and he are already at

When it comes to talking about sex, is your partner the silent type? If so, use these questions to pry his unspoken fellatio fantasies out of him. If he's the talkative type, these questions can still help you further refine your oral skills.

ease talking about your sex life, use these questions as catalysts to explore his wants and desires even more deeply.

Here are the questions:

1. Do you prefer fellatio as foreplay, the featured sex act, or both?
2. What are your favorite positions in which to receive fellatio?
3. Do you like it when I talk dirty before and during oral sex?
4. What are the most sensitive spots on your genitals?
5. Do you like me to pleasure myself as I perform fellatio?
6. What fantasy elements would you like to employ during oral sex?
7. What are your favorite ways to come when receiving fellatio?
8. Do you enjoy anal play?
9. Are you satisfied with our use of pornography, or do you want more?
10. What kinds of sex toys would you like to experiment with?

Printed in the United States
by Baker & Taylor Publisher Services

Printed in the United States
by Baker & Taylor Publisher Services

This his and hers guide to oral sex is full of fresh ideas and innovative techniques that are guaranteed to heat things up in the bedroom (or the kitchen, or the car, or…wherever the mood feels right!). Here are tips on:

- Verbal seduction (aka dirty talk)
- The art of the "full-body kiss"
- The sexiest body-massage techniques known to man and woman
- And, of course, mind-blowing oral sex

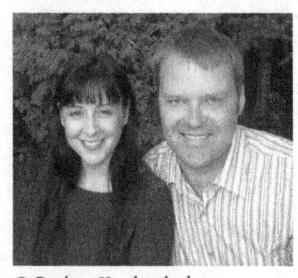
© *Darlene Vandenakerboom*

Don and Debra Macleod are the husband-and-wife authors of *Lube Jobs: A Woman's Guide to Great Maintenance Sex* and *The French Maid: And 21 More Naughty Sex Fantasies to Surprise and Arouse Your Man.*

A Man's Guide to

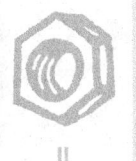

LIP SERVICE

the Art of Oral Sex and Seduction

Don and Debra Macleod

Jeremy P. Tarcher/Penguin

a member of Penguin Group (USA) Inc.

New York

Acknowledgments

Thank you to Joel Fotinos and Sara Carder for continuing to support our work. Thanks also to everyone at Tarcher, including Katherine Obertance for her first-rate editing, and Laura Ingman and Jennifer Levy for their publicity work.

As always, we extend our gratitude and friendship to Susan Raihofer, the literary agent of any writer's dreams. Your general brilliance and your ability to critique adult-rated proposals with such cool clarity, especially while riding the train, amaze us.

Contents

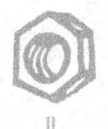 **LIP SERVICE**

Introduction: The Mouth as a Sexual Organ

Gentlemen, ask yourselves a question: What is your biggest sex organ?

Wrong.

Believe it or not—and eventually you will believe it—a man's most powerful, female-friendly sex organ isn't front and center between his legs; it's his mouth. Yes, yes, your penis is wonderful. The fullness of penetration and the friction of thrusting are feelings that most women find highly enjoyable. Yet there's a certain...um...attention to detail that only the mouth can deliver. The action of a man's tongue sliding over her clitoris or softly licking her labia can create intensely pleasurable sensations for a woman. If these actions are performed with skill, her pleasure is amplified.

Cunnilingus is an art, and as such it requires a certain amount of study and practice to be mastered. *Lip Service* makes it easy. Inside, you'll find all the information you need to master the art of oral sex, including female genital anatomy and issues and questions surrounding the practice of cunnilingus (such as "Why won't

she relax?" and "How can I get her to trim herself?"), as well as step-by-step practical techniques. You'll even learn how to modernize this ancient art by incorporating sex toys into your five-star performance.

Although cunnilingus is exquisitely pleasurable for a woman, the old bull's-eye approach to oral sex—blindly targeting the clitoris while ignoring other high-score zones—doesn't always get a woman's rivers flowing. After all, even the most delicious meal tastes better when preceded by an appetizer: It awakens the taste buds and builds anticipation for the mouthwatering main course. In the same way, foreplay is needed to seduce and adequately arouse a woman before your tongue can dish out its pleasure.

Foreplay comes in two forms in *Lip Service*. The first is verbal seduction. From sweet nothings to sinful somethings, you'll learn what, when, and how to say the things that will turn your woman on and make her eager for intimacy. Full-body kissing is the second form of foreplay. It is the ultimate erotic activity with which to seduce and arouse a woman, and it's guaranteed to hit the mark every time. As your mouth moves all over her body, lavishing kisses, licks, and sucks all over her bare skin, she'll melt into a highly sensual state where her mind and body can fully receive all the pleasures of cunnilingus. *Lip Service* teaches you how to perfect the art of full-body kissing by focusing on a woman's erogenous zones and concentrating on the kissing styles, techniques, and patterns that will best stimulate each erotic hot spot.

So, gentlemen, kudos to you for spending some time between

the pages of this book. Take our word for it; it's time well spent. Not only will you become the lover of your woman's dreams, but you'll most likely reap some giant rewards yourself. For once your woman discovers what your mouth is capable of, she'll be eager to return the favor.

1 | The Art of Verbal Seduction

n case you haven't noticed, women are verbal creatures. They easily talk two or three times as much as men—and that's on a quiet day. Add some kind of noteworthy event—anything from juicy girlfriend gossip to your chronic fashion failings—and she'll set out on a speaking spree that'll blow your mind if it doesn't blow your ears first. But it isn't all bad. Don't you appreciate the solitude when she's behind closed doors on hour two of a four-hour "girl-talk" call? There's an upside to everything.

Perhaps the biggest upside of a woman's love of language is the potential to exploit her passion for sexy purposes. Lusty language can be libido-enhancing for women and, if well spoken, a wonderful way to use your mouth as a sexual organ. That being said, "dirty talk" is a dialect that the fairer sex may require some time to get comfortable hearing. If you want to use it, you'll have to work up to it.

Temperature and Timing

When it comes to women, dirty talk is a question of degrees—
precisely how hot does she like it?—and a man must carefully
raise the temperature of his words until his partner feels drawn to
the heat but doesn't get burned. Timing is another important factor that, like the temperature, must be "just so" before a woman
will respond to dirty talk. Even the warmest words will cool off
if they're served too soon. For the man who wants to incorporate
dirty talk into his and his partner's sex life, the challenge is selecting the words and phrases that will best appeal to his woman and
then speaking them at those moments she will be most receptive.
This takes a little thought and a little more practice.

The Devil's in the Details

If your woman is like most, her day is full of a thousand details.
There's the stress of her job, the piles of laundry on the floor, the
kids' homework, the stack of bills on the counter, the phone calls
she has yet to return, and so on and so forth. It's true what they
say: A woman's work *is* never done. Chances are good that even
when her head hits the pillow, her mind will still be racing: Did
she program the coffee maker? What will she make for the kids'
lunch tomorrow? Was Wednesday's important meeting scheduled
for eleven a.m. or one p.m.?

　　Many women find these types of distractions very difficult to let
go of. Worse, they're passion slayers when they follow her to bed.

Any sparks of sexual interest or arousal she may have had earlier in the day or evening are most likely long gone by the time she actually crawls between the sheets, effectively snuffed out by her own preoccupied thoughts. And what if her man tries to talk dirty or initiate sex while she is in this unsexy frame of mind? Well, let's just say his chances of success aren't exactly stellar.

Sometimes, a man will interpret his woman's apparent lack of sexual response as a personal rejection and simply roll over and go to sleep. This interpretation isn't just unflattering, it's often inaccurate. Your timing may just be off, and your lady may just need a gentle push to make the transition from a demanding workday to a naughty nightlife. Instead of resigning yourself and her to a sexless state, why not put in some extra effort and try to reignite her libido? A tuned-in lover who is dedicated to his partner's pleasure can help a woman move from distraction to desire in a surprisingly short time.

Pillow ~~Talk~~ Listening

One of the easiest, most effective ways to slow down the pace of a busy day and to relax your partner's body and mind is to engage in a little pillow talk or, more correctly, pillow listening. Lay your head on the pillow with your face intimately close to hers, and simply listen to what your woman has to say. *Really* listen. Don't reach for the remote or the newspaper; don't check your voice mail; and don't fall asleep. Give her your undivided attention and let her unload whatever is on her mind. It isn't necessary to offer suggestions or solutions to her problems; your support is all she needs.

Be sure to maintain eye contact with your woman as she vents her day's stresses. This shows that you're focused on her entirely and strengthens your intimate connection. Smile softly to convey affection, and occasionally reach out to brush her cheek or stroke her hair. For women, these sweet gestures are laced with sexuality, so don't underestimate the eroticism of a simple touch.

Undercover Investigation

An easy way to practice great pillow-listening skills is to use the "dig deeper" technique. Snuggle under the covers and ask your woman a question. The question you ask depends on the type of talk you're having. If the conversation is deep, you can ask her something like, "Where do you see yourself in five years?" If the conversation is wading in the shallow end, you can ask, "Are there any movies you'd like to see?"

When your woman answers, simply dig deeper into her response to prompt further discussion on the topic and stay on a subject that is of interest to her. If she says she wants to be an associate at XYZ firm in five years, ask her what she anticipates that would be like or how it might impact her life. If she says she wants to see XYZ movie, ask her what it is about that movie or about the actors that interests her. Again, just listen as she speaks, and remember that with each word she says, she's distancing herself further from her day's stresses, worries, and distracting details.

This type of "conversational listening" technique is more than just an effective way to learn more about your woman; it also gives her a sense of priority. Women may love to talk, yet they spend

most of their time listening to and meeting other people's needs, whether it be a husband's, a child's, an employer's, or a friend's. By letting her talk about herself and her interests, you make her feel special, important, and validated. And the more you give her these types of feelings, the more she will feel drawn to you.

Laughter and the Libido

Listening to your woman and digging deeper into her feelings are great ways to clear her mind of distractions, draw her to you, and make her receptive to intimacy. Humor is another possibility, providing it's done right. After all, who isn't drawn to someone who makes us laugh? The trick to using humor as an aphrodisiac is to not go over the top. Remember that you're going for sexy, not slapstick.

"My wife and I were sitting in the middle of the living room floor, sharing a pizza and having a few drinks," recalls Bryce, thirty-six. "Things were going great. We were both totally relaxed. I was telling her about the practical jokes I used to pull on my little sister, and she was giggling like a schoolgirl. I kept moving closer to her, until we ended up lying together on the floor."

"It felt good to be laughing like that again," says Monica, thirty-eight, Bryce's wife of ten years. "We hadn't been getting along that well, but his stories were so funny that I wanted to be close to him. He'd tell me about a joke he pulled on his sister, and I'd double over laughing, especially since I know his sister and I could picture her reaction. We were having a great time." Monica suddenly draws an irritated breath. "Until the joke, that is."

"It was stupid," says Bryce. "I'd like to blame it on the drink,

but I hadn't had that much. It was just bad judgment. My buddies always laughed at that joke, so I thought Monica might think it was funny, too. Or maybe I just didn't think at all."

The joke in question—one that involved the resemblance between a mature woman's breasts and a tube sock with a ball in it—didn't have the same humorous effect on Monica as it had on Bryce's drinking buddies.

"I had been feeling sexy and confident," says Monica, "but that all changed as soon as he delivered the punch line. Instantly, I felt insecure about my body. I've had three kids; I'm almost forty; and I know my breasts are fighting gravity. The last thing I need is to hear a joke about it from my husband. To hear Bryce laughing about a woman's breasts made me tremendously self-conscious about my own. It made me angry, too, since I felt like I was getting mixed messages. On one hand he was turned off by a woman's breasts, but on the other he was trying to get a look at mine. In the span of five seconds, the fun, romantic mood was broken. I went to bed. Alone."

"I was shell-shocked," says Bryce. "I didn't know what hit me. One minute she's laughing; the next she's telling me to sleep on the couch. The joke was in poor taste and obviously the timing couldn't have been worse; but I didn't mean it the way she thought, that's for sure. Monica has a very sexy body, and I've always been attracted to it. It's taken a lot to undo the damage of that one stupid joke."

Learn from Bryce's mistake, boys. Save the adolescent sex jokes for the locker room, and stick to more tasteful material when you're wooing your woman. Humorous or entertaining anecdotes work well, whether drawn from your own experience or someone else's;

however, if your joke would sound great followed by a vaudevillian *ba-dum-ching* drum roll or if the listener usually reacts to the punch line with a grossed-out grimace, it probably isn't going to light up your woman's libido.

Mouth Maintenance

Congratulations! You've been an excellent listener, given your lady a laugh, and ushered her into a relaxed state where she's ready for more carnal conversation. Yet before you talk dirty, you need to get clean. Specifically, you need to ensure your oral hygiene is up to specs. Even the sweetest words will sound (and smell) foul if accompanied by coffee breath or, worse, scraps of the day's menu items lingering between yellow teeth or on grungy gums. Doesn't sound appetizing, does it?

Forgive us if it seems patronizing to point out the importance of good oral hygiene, but it's a necessity that warrants mention. All of us, particularly those of us tucked into comfortable long-term relationships, are guilty of occasionally overlooking the mouthwash before sliding under the sheets next to our significant other. There's no harm done if sleep is all that's on the agenda, but if you're hoping to stay up for a while, keep in mind that an unclean mouth can wreak havoc on a woman's desire.

Since your mouth is a powerful sex organ, maximize its efficiency by making sure it is as attractive as possible. You make sure your other sex organs are clean and tidy before use, don't you? Your mouth deserves the same level of maintenance. Have your teeth professionally cleaned on a regular basis, brush and floss

before snuggling next to your sweetie, and *always* use mouthwash when you're planning to get close, regardless of the "two-in-one" promises your toothpaste makes. You want your words to smell as fresh as they sound.

Sweet Nothings

The timing of the transition from warm-and-cozy pillow talk to hot-and-bothered passion talk is up to you. You know your woman best, so watch for the telltale signs that she's left her day's distractions in the dust and is now ready to heat things up: She may sigh, smile, flirtatiously snuggle closer to you, touch your body, and/or begin to use more suggestive language herself. Don't rush the process. Instead, wait for her cues before stepping up the action.

When the time is right to raise the temperature of your words, you can start slowly by whispering sweet nothings in your woman's ear. Sounds trite? Maybe, but trite or not, it is remarkably effective. Whispering sweet nothings works for a number of reasons. First, the suggestive sentiments you're verbalizing will make your woman feel attractive and aroused. Second, the closeness of your mouth and body is sexually stimulating. Third, the erotic sound quality of your whispers and the feel of your hot breath in her ear are highly sensual delights that will have most women swooning before you can finish your sexy sentence.

In regard to this last point, be aware of the volume and tone of your words as you sweet-talk your woman. You don't want to whisper so quietly that she must strain to hear you, but do speak in a hushed fashion. A male voice is typically deeper and lower

than a female's, and many women are turned on by the sound of a masculine voice caressing their ears. It's a sexy trait you come by naturally, so don't forget to make the most of it. For even greater impact, intersperse your breathy sentiments with light kisses or tongue flicks to your woman's ear, or gentle sucks on her earlobe.

Now that you recognize the passion punch those cliché sweet nothings can pack, you might be wondering what exactly *are* sweet nothings?

Flattery Will Get You Everywhere

For starters, flattery is a fantastic sweet nothing. It's easy, too, since all you must do to sing your woman's praises is tune that silver tongue of yours, and remember the three Ss of flattery: simplicity, sincerity, and sensuality. Keep your compliments simple and sincere: "Your eyes are lovely" sounds more heartfelt than "Your eyes are heavenly orbs of vibrant color and sparkling reflection." In the same way, "Your skin tastes so good," is more sensually flattering than a matter-of-fact "I like your skin."

Of course, your woman will love to hear how beautiful her eyes, hair, legs, breasts, and curves are, but don't limit yourself to flattering her appearance. Complimenting her on her character, abilities, accomplishments, or the way she makes you feel about yourself is also a touching way to flatter any woman. Compliments that focus on your woman's sexual desirability and lovemaking skills are perhaps the most erotic type of flattery you can dish out. As long as these types of compliments don't get too sexy too soon, they're a good way to segue into more sexual talk.

My girlfriend can't accept a compliment to save her life. If I tell her she looks nice, she says, "No, I don't," or acts like I'm just trying to butter her up for sex. How can I get her to believe me?

♀ *Debra*: Women are socialized to deflect and downplay compliments. Chances are, she's happy to receive your kind words but feels that accepting them will make her appear high on herself. Have a heart-to-heart with your girlfriend: Tell her that you enjoy complimenting her, that your compliments are sincere, and that it's frustrating when she contradicts you.

♂ *Don*: It took forever for Deb to just say "thank you" to a compliment. Until your girlfriend is more comfortable receiving compliments on her physical appearance, dish out compliments on her other attributes, such as her intelligence or sense of humor.

If you're still not sure what to whisper, try a few of these flattering yet frisky phrases as conversation openers:

- Your hair is so soft and smells so good.
- Your lips look delicious; I can't wait to taste them.
- You're so beautiful.
- I love looking into your eyes.
- All I could think about today was being close to you.
- How did I get such a smart, sexy woman in my bed?

- Your body is so soft, so smooth, it feels wonderful under my hands.
- Nobody makes me feel the way you do.
- I love the way you use your body in bed.

Memory Lane and the Libido

In addition to flattery, sweet nothings can include talk about romantic times you and your woman have shared. Nostalgia has a way of rousing emotions, so smile as you fondly reminisce about those special getaways, whether it was a luxurious honeymoon in Hawaii or a long-weekend campout in the woods. Revisiting your history as a couple helps strengthen your current bond and can really ramp feelings of sexual connection, particularly for women.

After you've relived your most loving moments, you can shift the focus to lustier memories, thereby bringing a more erotic tone to the conversation and paving the way for some down-and-dirty talk. Think about the raciest rendezvous you and your woman have enjoyed. Recall as many details as possible: Where were you? What did you or she do that pleasured the other so much? What position(s) were you in? Was there music playing in the background? Articulate the sexual feelings you experienced: You can tell her how intense your orgasm was, how wet she was, or how her nails dug almost painfully into your back. You can even tell her that you've masturbated to that mind-blowing memory. Remembering a past orgasmic experience can inflame the present libido, so go ahead and be a chatterbox.

The Woman of Your Dreams

Flattery and naughty nostalgia are great, but perhaps the sexiest way to seduce your partner with sweet nothings is to tell her that she's the woman of your dreams... your wet dreams, that is. When you tell a woman that she's in your dreams, you let her know that she has a place deep in your heart and mind. Better still for your purposes, you make her feel like the object of your sexual desire.

I love to talk dirty to my wife, and she likes to hear it. But she's tight-lipped and won't say a word. Do you have any ideas to loosen her up?

♂ *Don*: Before you ask her to talk dirty, just try to get her talking. When you're kissing or cuddling, ask her to tell you about her sexual fantasies. Get her to whisper innocent things before asking her to scream smut.

♀ *Debra*: Try appealing to her sympathies: Tell her that you love talking dirty but that you feel silly when it's a one-way conversation. Let her know how much more comfortable, and aroused, you'd be if she'd join in the conversation. And remember that many women aren't born with a dirty vocabulary. Give her a few ideas of what you'd like to hear, and make sure she knows such language won't make her any less "ladylike."

And when a woman feels wanted sexually, she is more confident, eager, and passionate.

As always, start out slowly and safely. A teasing approach works well. You can mischievously reveal that you had a sexual dream about her and then make her pry the details out of you. The harder she pries, the dirtier the details you provide. This not only builds anticipation but also lets your woman set the erotic pace. If she's game to get dirty, she'll keep digging in the mud.

Since you know your woman best and are privy to what she finds arousing, it is best if you dream up your own dreams. If you're not feeling imaginative, however, you can elaborate on these few flights of fancy:

- I dreamt that we didn't know each other. You hired me as a gigolo and told me to go down on you. You kept telling me what to do—suck softer, lick your clit, slide my finger inside—and I got so hard that I thought I was going to come.
- I dreamt that we were working out at the gym, and you left to go shower. I snuck into the woman's locker room and slipped into the shower with you. I knelt down and tongued you to orgasm. You had to be quiet so no one would hear.
- I dreamt that you tied my wrists to the headboard. You stood on the bed and stripped, and then lowered your pussy onto my mouth and told me to lick you. It was a delicious dream, and seeing you like that made me hard.
- I dreamt that we were undressing each other when we noticed that our bedroom window was open and our

neighbors were watching. You sat on the edge of the bed, and I knelt on the floor. I spread your legs and ate you out while they watched.

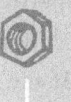 Don't cold-start dirty talk. Gradually raise the temperature of your words by whispering sweet words of flattery into your woman's ear and remembering the raciest romantic experiences you've shared. Segue into hotter talk by telling her you had a dirty dream about her.

Sinful Somethings

Now that you've warmed up your woman by whispering sweet nothings, you can set her arousal ablaze by uttering sinful somethings. Basically, you can begin to talk dirty. Yet how muddy the waters get will depend on your particular woman's comfort level and preferences. Does she like sensual language, or does she like it smutty? Would she respond better to desperate requests or to dominating commands?

Flipping through the pages of women's erotic fiction can give us an idea of what kind of words, phrases, and images fire up the female libido. There is a broad spectrum of sexual writing that's marketed for women, and it runs the gamut from petal soft to rock hard. Traditional, formulaic romance novels are on the tame side, often using words such as *his manhood* and *her depths*, and relying more on the romance angle than explicit language; however, the

growing genre of women's erotica is becoming ever more graphic, and many imprints are offering highly explicit reading for the modern woman. Words like *engorged cock* and *greedy pussy* are on the rapid rise. You need only check out a couple of our books to see on which side of the fence we fall.

Snoop in your woman's bedside drawer to see what kind of nighttime reading she has. Does the book jacket sport a long-haired airbrushed hero cradling a reluctant heroine in his trunklike arms? Or is the title something along the lines of *The Best Women's Smut on Earth*? If her bedside drawer is empty, march her off to the bookstore and escort her down the erotica aisle, telling her to choose some sexy bedtime reading material. It'll be a fun shopping trip for her and an instructional one for you.

Choose Your Words

Even though woman's erotica is getting raunchier all the time, it can still generally be distinguished from men's pornographic writing, which tends to be darker, more vulgar, and sometimes demeaning to women. You must therefore make the distinction between what you think is dirty talk and what your woman thinks it is.

The only way to be safe is to start slowly and to experimentally push the boundaries. As we've said, women are verbal creatures. They feel words as much as they hear them, and each word is loaded with meaning, imagery, and emotion. Words like *box*, *cunt*, or *bitch* may be basic dirty talk for some men, but for many women, these words are imbued with a sense of degradation. Your woman might be okay hearing these kinds of words at some point, but they

I said something during sex that I wish I could take back. I
told my wife of fifteen years that she fucks like a whore. I was
just trying to get her going, and I meant it in a good way, but
that's definitely NOT how she took it. How can I get out of the
doghouse?

♀ *Debra*: Wow, this is going to cost you. Literally. Take a trip
to the jewelry store, buy something sparkly, and present it to her
over a nice dinner out. Do it NOW. You have the security of a
fifteen-year marriage behind you, so that should mitigate your
misstep somewhat.

♂ *Don*: That's a tough one. When she lets you back in the house,
tell her what you *really* meant to say: that she's a gorgeous, lim-
ber, enthusiastic, exciting lover who blows your mind and that
she's more fun and sexy now than when you first met her.

should definitely *not* be in your starting lineup. Similarly, words
like *boobs* or *pecker* are insufferably adolescent. Keep in mind that
you're speaking to a grown woman, not a frat brat.

It may help if you think along these lines: Instead of just spout-
ing a dirty word, do your best to communicate an erotic idea, a
sexual sensation, or a provocative visual. Dirty talk isn't just about
spewing out obscene language. It's about giving your woman a
sexy image or feeling, or even a fantasy that she can play with in
her mind as you pleasure her body.

Instead of fretting over which specific dirty word(s) to say, focus on sharing a sexy idea or sensation. The words will flow more naturally. Also, remember the importance of sensual body language and eye contact as you speak.

Don't be afraid to discuss in advance which words your woman thinks will turn her on and which will turn her off. If this kind of conversation seems awkward, simply tell her that you want to talk about it beforehand out of respect for her. Dirty talk should fire up the libido, not extinguish it, and you don't want to say something offensive in the heat of the moment. By broaching this subject, you'll have given yourself some wriggle room and banked some forgiveness if you do accidentally put your foot in your mouth. In the same way, if you're in the middle of things and think you've overstepped, retreat and ask her directly if you spoke out of turn. A brief time-out is better than barreling forward if she has taken something the wrong way.

Scripted Sex Talk

Verbal seduction is fantastic foreplay to both full-body kissing and cunnilingus, so clear your throat and get ready to speak. Below, you'll find two short, sample sex scripts. The first is sensual; the second, smut. Chances are, your woman's linguistic preferences lie somewhere between these two poles. As you read each script,

make a mental note of the various words, phrases, and images you think would best arouse your woman. Don't try to memorize your lines. Sex talk isn't about studying; it's about seducing. Recited lines will sound unnaturally forced, so use these scripts as general guidelines. Use plenty of poetic license, and watch how your woman reacts to your words.

You should also keep in mind that the same expressions your woman may find distasteful on one occasion may appeal to her at another time, depending on her sexual mood. Revisit and revamp these scripts often, and, when your woman's mood seems especially adventurous, explore the R-rated version further.

Finally, be sure to use lots of body language as you speak. Look into your woman's eyes, and then hungrily gaze upon her body. If your words are romantic, lovingly stroke her hair, kiss her lips, and slip your hand under her PJs to physically stimulate her as your words mentally arouse her. If your words are raunchy, drag your fingertips hard over her bare skin, roughly press your body against her breasts, kiss her forcibly, and insistently position your leg or hand between her legs. Follow the script and do what's described, but don't hesitate to ad-lib and make your own director's cut.

G-Rated Romantic Ramblings

TIME: Nighttime.

SETTING: In bed or in the bath/shower.

YOU: I've been thinking about you all day, wishing I could be next to your naked body. Now that I am, I can feel my heart race and my

groin come alive. I can feel my body getting excited just by being close to you.

I love the curves of your hips, the way your breasts rise and fall as you breathe, the way you slightly part your legs when it's starting to feel good. It turns me on when I know you're feeling good.

I want to run my hands over your nakedness, over every inch of your body. I want to squeeze your nipples, taste them, and feel them get hard between my lips. I want to slide my hands up your legs, between them, and let my fingers graze over your wetness. I want to finger that little bud and hear you gasp, and then I want to slip my finger into your body, sliding it in and out until your wetness is running down your legs.

I want to explore your body with my mouth, too. Your lips, your neck, your shoulders, your breasts and nipples…they all feel different on my lips, they all taste different and delicious. The smoothness of your back always feels wonderful when I kiss it, so soft and womanly. I know you're sensitive there; I know how a long lick up your back can make your whole body shudder in anticipation of more. I know how a kiss on the back of your knees can make your juices flow.

I love the sight of your body below me, writhing in pleasure, eager for me to touch you again, desperate to feel my mouth licking, kissing, sucking. Your legs are so beautiful when they're wide open, presenting your most intimate place to my tongue. I'm so hard that it aches, but I know you want my tongue tonight. Your bud is so swollen. It can't wait to feel my tongue flick over it, circle it, suck it.

I can't wait, either. I can't wait to taste your juices and push my tongue deep into your body. I want to make you feel good tonight,

better than you've ever felt. I want your whole body to tremble, your legs to open wide, and I want my mouth to bring you to the strongest orgasm you've ever had. I love you so much.

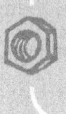

> I want to explore your body with my mouth...your lips, neck, shoulders, and breasts all feel and taste so different, so delicious, on my lips.

R-Rated Raunchy Ramblings

TIME: Anytime, day or night.

SETTING: Anywhere (bed, couch, car, hallway floor, closet).

YOU: Stay like that...don't move. You're going to take this. I've been thinking about grabbing your hair, holding your head still while I suck your tits until they're rock hard. You'd like that, wouldn't you? You'd like to feel my mouth assault you, my tongue snake into that tight pussy of yours. You'd like to feel my lips wrap around your clit and suck it until my face is wet from you. But I'm not going to make it that easy. I want to torment you, to hear you beg for it. And you will beg before I'm finished with you. You'll be begging me to stop, to give you release.

You act so innocent, but I know what you need even if you don't. You need to struggle. You need to feel your body burn with pain and pleasure. I'm going to make it hurt before it feels good.

Watch me work on you while I hold you down. Keep your eyes on me while my mouth bites and sucks at your body. Watch me as I lick your neck, drag my tongue down over your stomach toward your pussy. Sweet little sluts like you love to watch a man ravage them. They love to see a man's hot tongue leaving a wet trail over their skin. And they love the feel of a probing tongue teasing their clits, sliding along the lips of their pussy, and then invading them, torturing them. They love being helpless. But you'll have to wait for that. And beg. I like the taste of your flesh too much to release you that fast.

Roll over. I want to lick your back while my cock presses against your slit, but I won't put it in. As much as I'd love to fuck your pussy or your ass or your mouth, I'm not going to. I'm going to torture myself as much as I'm torturing you.

My mouth is going to make you come, not my cock. I'm going to tongue-fuck you until you beg me for release. Then I'm going to make you scream and spasm and tremble. Your pussy's going to clench around my tongue, and your orgasm is going to burn your body like a rush of fire.

Then I'm going to cream your body. While you're still squirming and groaning like a whore from your orgasm, I'm going to shoot thick streams of hot come on your tits or your stomach or your pussy. The heat of it on your bare skin is going to make your body climax again.

As you twitch beneath me, your pussy contracting and throbbing, begging for my tongue to come back, I'm going to squeeze the last drops of come out of my cock. And I'm going to watch as you rub it all over your body, making your skin glisten with it. You're going to love it.

> My mouth is going to make you come, not my cock.
> I'm going to tongue-fuck you until you beg me for
> release.

Raunch and Reassurance

A brief caveat about tough talk and rough sex: Know and respect your woman's sensibilities, boundaries, and reservations about these edgy sexual elements. Reassure her that dirty talk is simply a verbal expression of eroticism that you hope can amplify her arousal. In the same way, infusing your physical intimacy with a rough-and-tumble quality can bring an exciting new dimension to her oral-sex experience. If a woman is to enjoy this kind of bawdy behavior, she must know that it is an escapist, female-friendly way to increase her sexual pleasure and that it in no way reflects how you actually view her as a woman or as a lover.

Also bear in mind that while dirty talk is powerfully erotic in the throes of passion, its effect fizzles soon after orgasm. A word that sounded sexy a moment ago will suddenly sound silly. To ensure that your woman doesn't take sex talk too seriously, share a postorgasm laugh about your choice of language. It'll lighten the mood and help her realize it's all in fun.

Aural Arousal

It's a matter of record that many men love screamers. A woman who shrieks and gasps and yells with ecstatic abandon can really ramp a man's desire. This goes both ways: A man's low, deep, masculine voice is a natural turn-on for most women, particularly when he's whispering sinful somethings into her ear, but a man's loud sexual groans, heavy sighs, and throaty moans of pleasure can be even more stimulating. It reveals his manly, animalistic desire and makes her exquisitely aware of her own womanhood. If you find yourself lost for words in the throes of passion, feel free to remain speechless, as long as you still provide your woman with some aural arousal. Moan, groan, sigh, gasp, and desperately mutter her name, to demonstrate just how much you desire her.

Cat Got Your Tongue?

A final note about dirty talk: It's always better if it's a two-way conversation. Accordingly, do your best to draw your woman into the dialogue by asking her questions or otherwise prompting her to speak.

To bring your woman into the conversation, you can ask:

- Does it feel good when I kiss you here?
- Do you want me to keep doing this?
- Should I go softer or harder, slower or faster?
- Are you ready for me to lick you?

- Touch my cock...can you feel how hard this is making me?
- Do you want me to stop?
- Am I doing it good?
- Should I kiss you here or there?
- Can you feel your orgasm building?
- What can I do to make you come right now?

Since *Lip Service* uses dirty talk as a form of foreplay to full-body kissing and cunnilingus, you can use this very intimate form of discourse to learn all you can about your woman's body, including how to best pleasure it. That way, your skills will be second to none when you practice these erotic arts.

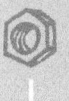 Lost for words? Moan, sigh, or gasp. The sounds of a man's pleasure are arousing to a woman. Is your lady tight lipped in bed? Draw her into a dirty dialogue by asking questions like "Should I go faster or slower?" or "Are you ready for me to lick you?"

If your partner is on the shy side, getting her used to hearing and speaking erotic language is also a great way to increase your sexual communication in a broader sense, as a couple. Once you've done that, you and she will be able to discuss your sex life, including your desires and dislikes, in an easy and open manner. Your tongue can't be put to better use.

2 | Female "Feel-Good" Zones

O f all the chapters in *Lip Service*, this one may be the most important. In fact, it should be required reading for all men. Women are sexy creatures, and their bodies are capable of receiving, and responding to, intense erotic pleasure that goes far beyond vaginal or clitoral stimulation. Yet it is remarkable how many men, even very sexually experienced men, don't realize the full-body bliss they could be giving their partners.

Men must realize that a woman's sexuality, including her body's erogenous or "feel-good" zones, is multilayered. As a man learns to peel back each layer, he gets ever closer to providing his partner with the ultimate mind/body sexual experience.

The Feeling of Femininity

Despite what you may think, a woman's primary feel-good zone isn't a physical location on her body; it's an emotional state of mind. Before a woman can really enjoy physical pleasure, she must feel emotionally

confident in her sexual desirability. Just as a man likes to have his sexual ego stroked, a woman likes to feel that her natural femininity is noticed and admired. This doesn't translate to gawking at or grabbing her breasts. Rather, it involves a man appreciating all of her womanly attributes, including those that take a backseat to those bra-clad show stealers. Your lady's overlooked attributes may include:

Her face: What woman doesn't like to be told that she's beautiful to her man? Outline her face with your fingertips while you tell her how lovely she is to you.

Her hair: Brush her hair and run your fingers through it, noting how soft it feels, how good it smells. Women spend tons of time (and money!) on their manes, so provide her a payoff by caressing and complimenting it.

Her figure: Running your hands over your partner's body while you openly admire her womanly curves can really make her feel sexy. Don't focus on any body part in particular; just show her that you love her figure, be it full or frail.

Her movements: Even if your woman is an accident waiting to happen, make sure you emphasize how graceful you find her movements both in and out of bed.

Her voice: Noticing a woman's sexy voice makes her feel feminine from within. Smile when she speaks or sighs to let her know how much the sound of her lusty but lovely voice turns you on.

She's in Your Hands

In the woman's guide version of *Lip Service*, we make the distinction between a man's pleasure zones and his erogenous zones. Pleasure zones are those areas of a man's body that simply feel pleasant when they're stimulated, such as his back or his feet. Erogenous zones are those areas that lead to an erotic response when stimulated, such as the glans of his penis or his testicles. But when it comes to women, the pleasure/erogenous distinction is often an artificial one. This is due to the multilayered nature of female arousal. For that reason, we've grouped them together as "feel-good" zones.

For example, what begins as a basic back rub that feels pleasant to a woman may quickly morph into a sensual massage that feels erotic. The difference—and your woman's arousal—is in your hands. If your technique is lackluster and you just dutifully squeeze her shoulders, her libido probably won't kick in; however, if your technique is lustful and you let your hands sexily roam, her libido will likely respond.

Because of a woman's physical sensitivity, every inch of her body has the potential to be an erogenous zone. Keep that in mind as you study the following areas of the female form, and try to shake the male misperception that it's only a woman's genitals that are worth stimulating. The truth is, her clitoris and vagina should be the last items on your list. If you can learn how to excite her entire body first, you'll find that her genitals are more ready and responsive than ever. A woman's feel-good zones are many and

multilayered, and a knowledgeable lover knows how to stimulate them all in turn.

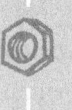

> It isn't just your woman's genitals that you need to stimulate. In truth, her clitoris and vagina should be last to receive erotic attention. If you excite her entire body first, her genitals will be ready for and responsive to your touch.

Female Feel-Good Zones

Your woman's feel-good zones may include:

Her scalp: Massaging and/or scratching your woman's scalp will stimulate blood circulation, which feels good and dissolves distractions.

Her face: A tender caress over your woman's eyelids and cheeks can rouse very special feelings of intimacy.

Her lips and mouth: Stroking your woman's lips with your fingertips and kissing her mouth are sweet, simple ways to say "I love you. I desire you." A kiss is also a promise of more to come, and it can make a woman's desire start to smolder. Like the lips, the tongue is also an erogenous zone: Stimulate her tongue with your own to increase eroticism, anticipation, and sexual response.

Stimulating the frenulum (the flap of tissue that connects the upper lip to the gums) may also turn on your woman.

Her ears: The ear area is packed with bundles of nerve endings that make them extremely sensitive. The earlobe, flap, and canal are highly responsive to erotic stimulation such as sucking, licking, nibbling, breath blowing, whispering, tongue penetrating, and so forth. The area behind the ear is also very sensitive, particularly as it leads down to the sides of her neck, another feel-good zone.

Her neck: A woman's exposed neck is as sexy as it is vulnerable. Think of those vampire movies—Dracula's always enticing, isn't he? Well, your woman thinks so. Perhaps it's this element of instinctual, animalistic danger that makes neck stimulation so sexually arousing. The sides of your woman's neck, the front, and the nape of her neck all respond strongly to erotic contact, whether it's kissing, nibbling, or stroking.

Her breasts, areola, and nipples: The breasts are ultrasensitive feel-good zones that should be thought of in three parts: the fleshy mound of breast, the areola (the pigmented area around the nipple), and the nipple. Stimulation of each distinct part gives your woman a uniquely arousing sensation, so give each area the attention it deserves. The nipples in particular are highly erogenous, and proper treatment (at the right time, with the right pressure) can lead to a strong sexual response.

Her inner arms, inner elbows, wrists, and palms: The skin on the inner arm, including the inner elbow, is thin and sensitive,

making these areas ripe for stimulation. Similarly, the inner wrists and the palm are oft-neglected spots that respond well to touch, be it a lick, kiss, or fingertip caress.

Her sides: The stretch of skin alongside your woman's body—from her armpits/sides of her breasts, down to her hips—is a large, very sensitive erogenous zone that reacts sexually to stroking, licking, kissing, and so on. The side of the body is an area that isn't normally touched in a tender way (think of your poor lady sandwiched on the elevator at work, her sides serving as bumpers against fellow occupants), and this may be one reason the area appreciates a softer touch.

Her navel area: Your woman's navel area—from her belly button to about where her pubic hair begins—is a feel-good zone not only because it's sensitive but also because it leads the way to her genitals. Perhaps because of its proximity to the womb, this area can be a very sweet and special place to caress a woman. It is closely tied in to her femininity.

Her inner thighs: Like the sides of her body, your woman's inner thighs are areas that don't normally receive a lot of stimulation. They therefore respond quickly to erotic contact. The inner thigh's proximity to the groin is another reason. It's hard to stimulate the inner thigh without grazing the genital region, whether it be with a brush of your hair or arm, or the feel of your breath, and the inadvertent contact causes spikes of intense sexual expectation.

Her feet: You might regularly rub your woman's shoulders and back, but how often do you treat her tired feet to a massage? Yeah, we thought so. A foot rub is a sumptuous, sexy indulgence for a woman to experience, so give your woman a taste of this delicacy. Who knows? Maybe you'll both uncover a hidden foot fetish.

Her shoulders and back: Because your woman carries a great deal of her tension in her shoulders and back, these areas provide a large canvas on which you can work to relax her via a variety of massage techniques. More important, these areas are supercharged with sexual sensation. Caressing a woman's shoulders and back with touches, strokes, licks, and kisses is almost certain to arouse her body and mind. So the next time you're having trouble stimulating your woman, stop what you're doing and begin to lavish her shoulders and back (all the way from the nape of the neck to the lower back, just above the buttocks) with sensual touch. She'll come around.

Her buttocks: Like the back, the buttocks provide a large surface area of sexually charged sensation. Lightly gliding your palms over her buttocks can summon very sensual thoughts and feelings. Squeezing them can rouse more desperate desire. Many women enjoy spanking and find that it leads to an even more intense effect. Spanking increases blood flow to the buttocks that many women enjoy for both the mental aspect as well as the physical burn. For the woman who enjoys anal play, stimulating the buttocks makes her anticipate anal contact.

Her anal area: Your woman's anal area is loaded with nerve endings and is exceptionally responsive to sexual stimulation, both outside and inside. That being said, there are many cultural forces and perceived taboos that may prevent your woman from letting you explore this erogenous zone. The topic of anal play is covered in later chapters (particularly chapters 5, 6, 8, 9, and 10).

Her genitals: Your woman's genitals are the most sensitive and intensely powerful erogenous zones on/in her body, the ones directly involved in orgasm. Her genitals boast a number of distinctly powerful hot spots, from her labia and clitoris to her perineum and G-spot, that can provide unparalleled pleasure. The specific location of these hot spots, as well as ways to stimulate them, will be discussed in later chapters (particularly chapters 6, 8, 9, and 10).

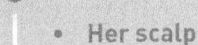 **Her feel-good zones at a glance:**

- Her scalp
- Her face, including her lips, mouth, and ears
- Her neck
- Her breasts, areola, and nipples
- Her inner arms/elbows, wrists, and palms
- Her sides and her navel
- Her inner thighs
- Her shoulders, back, and buttocks
- Her anal area
- Her genitals

Again, even though the genitals are the most powerful erogenous zones on/in a woman's body, they should be the final feel-good zones to be stimulated. It is only when a woman's body and mind are in a state of arousal that the genitals are receptive to touch. Attempting to stimulate a woman's genitals too soon, before she is sufficiently turned on, is unpleasant for a woman. In fact, it's probably the leading mistake that men make when trying to arouse their women.

The Dash versus The Detour

"I used to be known as Mad Dash Max," says Max, thirty-six. "I always thought it was a kind of compliment, until I overheard my girlfriend talking on the phone to a friend. She was complaining about how I just dove for her clit without warming her up first. It was then that I clued in to what "Mad Dash Max" really meant. It wasn't a compliment."

Happily, Max has since changed his ways. And it's his wife, Liv, who has reaped the benefits of his personal sexual reformation.

"I call him Mad Detour Max now," says Liv. "He doesn't make a mad dash for anything anymore. Now he takes his time and makes a lot of stops along the way. I have nothing to complain about."

"I've really changed how I think about a woman's body," Max explains. "I don't just head straight for the genitals. Instead, I think of all her erogenous zones as destinations. I take a detour to each one before I touch her pussy or clit, or even her nipples. By the time I get to those spots, she's squirming and already very wet. It's way better than fingering a dry clit and praying for rain."

Max has it right, gentlemen. Slow down and take plenty of detours around your woman's body, exploring all of her feel-good zones before zeroing in on her genitals. Barring those spontaneous up-against-a-wall quickies where she's already aroused, your woman needs some time to warm up before she can get hot.

3 | Setting the Mood

So...your wife's just put dinner in the oven, the television's blaring, and the kids are fighting at her feet. Or maybe your girlfriend just got home from a bad day at work, her car broke down, and the dry cleaner lost her little black dress. Let's think for a moment, boys. Is this *really* the time to try and tweak her nipples? The importance of timing and setting the mood can't be emphasized enough when it comes to sexually prepping a woman. Doesn't her collection of scented candles betray how important a sensual atmosphere is to her?

The art of oral sex and seduction isn't just about learning a new mouth move or tongue twist. It's also about bringing your woman to a pure, heightened state of arousal where she can fully experience the erotic power of your mouth as a sexual organ. Verbal seduction and knowledge of her body's feel-good zones are fundamental to the mental and physical stimulation of your woman, but before you can put what you know into practice and perform a full-body kiss and cunnilingus, you must set the mood—and get her in the mood—for these erotic events.

Sex and the Senses

During an intimate encounter, a man's body engages all five of a woman's senses—sight, sound, smell, touch, and taste—to varying degrees. The way a man moves and prepares his body can therefore create an enticing aura. Your body has the potential to be a sensorial delight to your woman, so always be mindful of the following points.

TOUCH The feel of a man's skin, muscles, and strength, moving and pressing against her body is a powerful turn-on for a woman. To exploit your natural manliness, grow a beard and graze your woman's bare skin with it; if you already have a beard, shave it to let her delight in the unfamiliar feel of your smooth face.

SIGHT It's a well-known fact that men are visually stimulated, but don't be fooled; women love the sight of a man's sexy body working its wonders on her. Accordingly, play with what nature gave you by sometimes shaving, sometimes trimming, and sometimes letting your pubic hair go au naturale. If you're game, you can also wax your chest or body hair to let her see you in a different way.

TASTE To add yum to your kisses, always use mouthwash before initiating sexual activity. If you're going to be engaging in mutual oral sex, watch your diet beforehand and avoid alcohol, red meat, and dairy products, since these can make semen distasteful. Chow down on fruits and vegetables instead. Also, practice good personal hygiene by washing your genitals before asking your woman

to put them in her mouth (this is especially important if you're uncircumcised).

SOUND As discussed in chapter 1, The Art of Verbal Seduction, sexual expressions and sounds can increase a woman's desire. Remember the lessons of that chapter and use your word choice and tone as well as your moans, sighs, and the rhythm of your breathing to set an erotic mood for intimacy.

SMELL If you're in a long-term relationship, you might've stopped using cologne a while back. Or maybe you've been splashing on the same drugstore brand since high school. Either way, buy yourself a new, high-quality men's fragrance. Your woman will love it. And again, if mutual oral sex is on the menu, make sure your equipment is squeaky clean and odor free. If you're tempted to spray your new cologne "down there" in the hopes of enticing her south, stop yourself; cologne smells good but tastes awful.

> Your body can be a sensorial delight to your woman, so do your best to engage all of her five senses—sight, sound, smell, touch, and taste—during sex.

Location and Lip Service

It's no secret that a beyond-the-bedroom-walls sex session can set the mood for an exciting event. Yet when it comes to body kissing and oral sex, many women don't share the same wandering tendencies

as their male counterparts. Sure, a quickie blow job in the front seat of the car (or in the closet, under the table, even hanging from the ceiling) is an easy enough accomplishment for you, but many women need a more relaxed, comfortable location to enjoy receiving cunnilingus.

That's not to say a woman can't enjoy a spontaneous or speedy encounter. In fact, a great many women thrive off them. You know your woman; so you be the judge. Yet it may be best, at least initially, to perform full-body kissing and oral sex in a location where your woman feels at ease. The bedroom and the bathroom are obvious choices because of their private, richly sensual atmospheres.

When you're ready to branch out of the bedroom/bathroom, why not simply slide onto the floor? A change of location doesn't have to be anything radical, since it's the elements of variety and unfamiliarity that make the experience thrilling, not the different color on the walls. Even the hallway floor can be a sexy place to perform full-body kissing and oral sex. The rough carpet under your naked bodies, the strangeness of being on the ground, the close walls, and the sense of exhibitionism all combine to make an in flagrante floor coupling an exciting alternative to the boudoir.

> A change of sexual location doesn't have to be radical; it's the elements of variety or unfamiliarity that make the experience thrilling.

Once your woman has shed any lingering inhibitions and can let herself go, you can give it to her anytime, anywhere. Remember

that dirty dream where she was the main course at a sex supper? Clear the kitchen table and lay her body on top to make that dream come true. And what about that oh-so-comfy reclining, vibrating easy chair in the living room? Settle her bare body between those arms and put that real leather to good use. Finally, don't forget the great outdoors; sex under the stars is absolute heaven.

Passion Props and the Power of Erotica

Passion props are anything you use to help set the stage—and the mood—for an unforgettable oral-sex experience. (This doesn't include the use of sex toys, which is the subject of chapter 9.) In the women's guide, we suggest the use of such things as mirrors, bright lighting, and pornography, all things that appeal to the "visual" male. While many women do enjoy these things, they also delight in a softer approach. For example, dim lighting, romantic music, and audio erotica (CDs of couples having sex) can really set a sensual mood for a woman.

Erotic literature is one of the best passion props you can use to get your woman in the mood for sex, since erotic writing has a powerful effect on the female libido. If you don't believe us, think about the annual earnings of the romance publishers. For the lady who doesn't like porn, written erotica is a great alternative. For the woman who does watch XXX, the verbal, imaginative quality of erotica is an alluring adjunct to visual porn. It's all about variety.

We've included three supershort, supersexy erotic stories that you can have your partner read or, even better, read aloud to her. Each story features a woman as the central character (don't take it

personally; this is about her!) enjoying a provocative sexual experience. You can expect that, after your woman turns the last page of this frisky fiction, she'll be turning to you for the real thing.

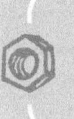

> To fire up her libido, have your woman read the following supershort, supersexy erotic stories. Better yet, read them aloud to her.

The Total-Body Treatment

It had been ages since she'd had a massage, but after enduring a two-week visit from her mother-in-law, Madeline knew she had earned the luxury. She lay facedown on the massage table, listening to the relaxing mood music, letting the lavender aromatherapy candle soothe her spirits and feeling the clean, crisp coolness of the sheets under her bare breasts. Pure heaven.

With her eyes closed, she heard Justin, the masseur, enter the room quietly. She had received a great massage from him a while ago and had specifically requested him again. Seeming to sense her stress, Justin said a hushed "hello," lowered the lights, and took a bottle of lavender-scented massage oil from a tray on the counter. She could smell its essence the moment he removed the cork from the glass bottle. Opening her eyes to return his greeting, Madeline was surprised to see another man in the room. He was young, maybe in his mid-twenties, dressed in the same white spa shirt as Justin.

"I have a massage student with me today," said Justin in that

same hushed tone. "His name is Jack. Do you mind if he participates or would you prefer not?"

"That's fine," said Madeline.

"Excellent," Justin replied with a soft smile.

Again, Madeline closed her eyes and focused on relaxing her mind and body. One of the masseurs lifted the sheet off her back and she enjoyed the feel of the air against her skin. The masseur folded the sheet down—far down—until it barely covered her buttocks. For a moment she felt a flare of vulnerability, but in the next moment, the oiled hands sliding up her back, untying the deep knots that gripped it, consumed her. It felt good.

The masseur's strokes were deep and long, moving up from her lower back to the nape of her neck. But as he kneaded her shoulders, she felt his warm breath in her ear and tensed at how unexpectedly close his face was to her body. "Relax and let yourself feel it," Justin—or was it Jack?—whispered, noticing her reaction. "Breathe into it."

Madeline felt the masseur's warm breath move down the back of her neck, down her spine to her lower back and shuddered again as she visualized his mouth only inches away from her bare skin. She felt the sheet move down her legs and off her body. She was naked.

Stunned at the suddenness of it and feeling heart-pounding vulnerability, she lay frozen with shock and uncertainty: Had the sheet fallen off accidentally? But then she felt strong, oiled hands on the back of her legs, confidently moving upward and upward. It was no accident. She swallowed hard as the masseur's hands slid up the back of her thighs... and didn't stop. She felt his thumbs graze her pussy, and instantly she felt an ache, moisture, and a longing to feel it again.

In a halfhearted act of protest, Madeline raised her head slightly off the massage table. Justin gently pushed it back down. "Close your eyes and don't open them until we're finished," he instructed gently. "We're going to gather all the erotic energy in your body, and then we're going to release it."

The ache swelled into a constant throb, and the moisture began to show on the sheets. Madeline suppressed a moan of profound pleasure and erotic anticipation as she felt four hands urging her to turn over, to expose her breasts and her pussy to their touch. She obeyed almost against her will and again delighted in the feel of the air against her bare skin, but this time was better as the elements of surrender and exposure amplified her senses.

She kept her eyes closed. One man stood above the mounds of her breasts; the other stood over her exposed patch of pubic hair. Their hands moved over her body, roaming, exploring, squeezing, and caressing. Her hips were moving on the table, and her skin was pink with flush. Madeline didn't need to see her nipples to know that they were tight and long. She felt a palm sweep over one of them and heard a gasp escape her lips. She felt the back of a hand brush against the wet, swollen lips of her pussy and her legs opened involuntarily.

She was struck hard by an onslaught of erotic sensation as one of the men gently pinched both of her nipples, while at the same time the other man spread her labia apart and lightly tapped her exposed clitoris. It sent a bolt of pleasure that made her body visibly shudder. She heard the men exchange soft sounds of approval. Her hips began to move more. Embarrassed, she tried to stop herself, but she was past that point. Needing more, she gyrated her hips shamelessly and arched her back, urging the masseurs to keep going.

They responded. The man above her breasts plucked her nipples tightly and pulled them until they were even longer. Then he stopped pinching them and leaned over to lick the hard, almost painfully elongated buds with the tip of his tongue. The man over her pussy tapped her clit faster and harder, spreading her further apart. Madeline felt his middle finger exploring her, probing for her entrance.

As the masseur's long finger sank into her, she let out an audible groan and bucked her hips off the table. His middle finger pivoted inside her and then stroked her internally, raking her G-spot. A strange, deep tremble of pleasure shook her inside and then spread to the surface of her body. The sheet was soaked. She felt the beginnings of an orgasm forming, and she knew it would be unbelievably strong. The anticipation was agonizing.

The long middle digit inside her body stroked her G-spot again, and then the tip of the masseur's tongue unexpectedly flicked over her raw clit. His tongue teased her clit, and then his mouth pressed against her pussy to suck it and taste her wetness. His middle finger began to thrust into her, in and out, fucking her. And then it was two fingers inside, making her feel full, fucking her more insistently, and expertly bringing her close to orgasm.

Seeing how close she was, the masseur over her breasts pinched and pulled her nipples hard for a moment and then stopped. His mouth came down on one breast and his lips sucked her nipple in rhythm with the man who was sucking her clit and finger fucking her pussy.

Not caring how she looked or what they thought, Madeline abandoned herself to the experience. Her body's most sensitive spots—her nipples, her pussy, her deep G-spot, and her clit—were

all being stimulated at the same time, her nervous system firing flares of unrelenting pleasure over and through her body. Her mind was empty, but her body was full of their fingers and tongues.

Their rhythm was irresistible, and her body fell into it. As the one masseur pumped his two fingers inside her body, tonguing her clit with each thrust, the other masseur sucked one nipple with his mouth, pinching the other between his fingers. Madeline's body matched their rhythm as her orgasm swirled into being like a tornado gaining strength. Her hips moved to accept the one man's long fingers into her pussy, and her back arched to push her breasts against other man's mouth.

Her mounting orgasm swirled faster until it formed completely and then burst apart, sending waves of almost painful sexual release over her hot skin and through her body. Madeline's body tensed as the cycle of her orgasm gripped her. She couldn't move, couldn't cry out, couldn't stop the men from pumping and tonguing and sucking as her orgasm pulsed and paralyzed her.

And then it was over. The intensity of her orgasm ebbed away, and in its place a feeling of calm and contentment flowed into her body. The masseurs thanked her and left the room, leaving her to dress in bewildered bliss.

She couldn't wait for her mother-in-law's next visit.

The Rendezvous

Jackie sat on the edge of the bed in the hotel room and stared emotionless at the wall in front of her. She knew she shouldn't

be there. If she had any sense, she'd stand up and walk out of the room before he arrived. It wasn't too late. She could still remain the faithful wife.

But then she heard the faint *click* of the hotel room door and turned her head to watch him enter the room. The door closed behind him, and he stood uncertainly across the room from her, the two of them looking at each other, feeling the tension mount and wondering what the other was thinking—as if they didn't know.

"I wasn't sure you'd come," Connor whispered hoarsely. "I'm glad you did."

She said nothing but looked back at the wall and blinked.

He wrung his hands. "You look good." He closed the distance between them and, cautiously, sat next to her on the edge of the bed. "I missed you."

"I missed you, too," Jackie admitted. She faced him, and they studied each other yet again, each enthralled by the other's closeness.

Connor lifted a hand and brushed it against her cheek. "I want you," he whispered, his voice even hoarser than before. "I've wanted you for so long."

"This is wrong," Jackie protested. But it was a weak protest, one she didn't have the strength to pursue. She knew she'd regret it when it was over, but at this moment she couldn't summon the will to refuse him or to leave or even to resist his mouth as it moved toward hers. A thousand times she had fantasized about kissing that mouth. "I want you, too," she said, her cracking voice betraying her inner conflict.

He saw her struggle and pulled back. "I don't want you to regret this," he said. "We'll take it slow. We'll see what happens." When she did not respond, he leaned in and kissed her lips. Growing

ever more excited, he sucked her tongue and felt the breath leave her body. "Let's take a shower."

Connor's words struck like a bolt of pleasure between her legs. She had a vision of their naked bodies pressed together in the sinful, secret space of the shower: wet, moving, and entwined, hidden from the eyes of her husband. Her clit began to pulse with expectation, swelling and moistening her panties.

He took her hand, and Jackie followed him across the room into the bathroom. The lights were dim. Connor reached into the shower and turned the water on. Within a few moments, the small room was hot and humid. Jackie's chest tightened and her stomach dropped as Connor's hands began to unbutton her shirt. He pushed it off her shoulders and, his movements becoming more eager, unfastened her bra. Staring lustfully at her breasts, he undressed himself as she stepped out of her skirt and panties.

Together, they stepped into the shower. As the warm water fell over their bodies, they gazed upon each other's nakedness, relishing the sight they had waited so long to see yet still were afraid to touch. Jackie stared at his length and felt her heartbeat quicken as it stiffened before her eyes. Slowly, Connor reached out and pressed his hand against her breast. She felt her nipple tingle and harden against his palm.

"I want to wash you," he said throatily and, taking a handful of body wash, spread it over her neck, shoulders, breasts, and stomach. He reached down to feel between her legs, washing her pussy until the suds mixed with her juices and ran down her legs. "Wash me," he said and poured some of the body wash into her hands.

Jackie closed her hands around his erection and spread the body wash along the hard, silky skin of his shaft, reeling from the

electric effect of his fingers as they washed and probed her labia. His fingertips slipped just inside her tightness, and in response to the invasion she tightened her clasp and began to pump him, feeling the swollen mushroom head of his cock pop in and out of her fist.

Connor had waited too long for this release, and he couldn't hold back. With another few strokes, he squeezed his eyes closed, and his loud groan echoed off the shower walls. He thrust into her fist, and the come jetted out of him in spurts of hot pleasure. Yet even after his orgasm, his cock seemed to lose none of its eagerness.

Breathing hard, he clutched Jackie's shoulders and directed her to sit on the tiled seat in the corner of the shower. She obeyed his every direction like an automaton. Once she was seated, Connor spread her legs wide and knelt between them. He retrieved a loofah sponge from a shelf and began to drag it over her bare skin. The slight scratching sensation raised goose pimples on her thighs.

Seeing the effect, Connor lowered his head and kissed her inner thighs. Jackie looked down at his head between her legs and then pressed her back against the coolness of the shower tile in an effort to ground herself. His mouth moved along one of her inner thighs and then the other before he raised his head and kissed her stomach, sliding his tongue inside her navel. As his tongue thrust into her navel, he slid the loofah along her pussy. Jackie lost her breath as the scratchy texture of the sponge razed her clit.

"Stop, that's too much," she gasped.

"I'll give you too much," he replied. And with that, his mouth was at her pussy. His tongue darted in and out of her, lapped her labia with a single long lick and then fluttered over her clitoris. He kissed her pussy like he had kissed her mouth, caressing the wet folds and then sucking on her clit like it was her tongue. He lifted

his head and sucked each of her nipples in the same way, before returning to her twitching clit.

His tongue thrust into her again and again, fucking her. Jackie felt his wet fingers separate her aching labia, spreading her open so that he could see her secrets. She felt the strong tip of his tongue trace each and every fold of flesh in her pussy. His tongue slid into her again, deeper than she imagined it could have, and she felt its thick fleshiness moving inside her. She felt an unbearable tingling, then a tugging, as his lips closed around her clit and he sucked again, as if trying to pull the tiny bud into his mouth.

Still sucking and tonguing her clit, Connor pressed two of his knuckles against Jackie's slit. She longed to feel something hard plunge into her body, but instead the pressure remained just at the entrance. It filled her body with an acute sense of anticipation. Each time Connor sucked on her clit, sparks of pleasure shot over her skin, directly to her nipples. The water cascaded down over her, and as each drop assaulted her hard nipples, she prayed that her body would give her the release of climax.

Suddenly, the water began to come down with more force, the beads of water hitting her nipples harder and harder until they hurt. Connor had increased the pressure. The combination of his sucks on her clit and the water pounding on her nipples was too much, and Jackie pressed the back of her head against the tile wall as the rush of orgasm began to flood her body.

Her orgasm came in sharp, sporadic currents of sensation. She gripped Connor's head and ground her pussy against his face, hoping he wouldn't stop sucking until the feeling had lost its intensity. He didn't. It was perfect. He seemed to instinctively know her body: It was like he had pleasured her a thousand times.

Connor pulled her to her feet, and they embraced under the warm rain of the shower. Together, they stepped out of the shower and wrapped themselves in towels. Finding his pants on the floor, Connor dug through the pockets and pulled out two wedding bands. He slipped one on his finger.

"Here's yours," he said with a wry grin.

"Thanks," replied Jackie, smiling and slipping the ring onto her finger. "There's nothing more thrilling than an affair, is there?"

"As long as it's with your husband," Connor happily confirmed.

The Wall Flower

Lily balanced herself against the wall. The music was pounding; the room was crowded; and her head was starting to spin. She poured the rest of her wine into a potted plant and set the glass on a bookshelf. It had been years since she'd been to a house party as wild as this one. Come to think of it, it had been years since she'd been to *any* party. Feeling slightly better, she leaned against the wall and watched the festivities. Couples were dancing and drinking. Singles were preening and prowling. The singles, except for her, that was. She smoothed the front of her skirt and sighed.

No wonder she was alone; the quintessential wall flower, Lily had bolted for the nearest escape route when a man—his name was Jeremy, and he had seemed harmless enough—had approached her. She felt like hitting her head on the wall. Why had she reacted so weirdly? Why couldn't she just stay and chat him up like the other women did so effortlessly? She scanned the room and spotted him

by the television. An attractive woman in a low-cut tank top was in the full throes of shameless flirtation, flicking her long curls, licking her collagen-enhanced lips, and strategically touching his arm.

Dejected, Lily watched the mating ritual. The woman was really strutting her stuff now. She laughed loudly and tossed her head back, placing a hand on her padded breasts to draw attention to them. Lily was still watching when the man unexpectedly looked in her direction and caught her eye. He smiled warmly and raised his glass to her. The padded woman followed his gaze and, when she noticed Lily, quickly took his arm and tried to escort him to another area of the room.

Lily's pulse quickened as the man, Jeremy, politely extracted himself from the woman's clutches and strolled across the room toward her. She forced herself to return his casual smile as he leaned against the wall next to her.

"Thought I had lost you in the crowd," he shouted over the music.

"No such luck," Lily shouted back.

"Wanna find someplace quieter?"

Lily fought the urge to bolt. "Sure."

Jeremy placed his empty glass next to hers on the bookshelf and took her hand. Lily felt her cheeks redden as his warm, strong hand led her out of the room, down a long hall, and into a small, secluded den. He closed the door behind them.

"Have you been here before?" Lily asked. "You seem to know this house."

"It's my brother's place. I used to live here with him before I moved out of town."

"So you're just visiting?"

"Yep," said Jeremy. "Just in town for a few cheap thrills," he added with a grin.

Lily tensed. His demeanor had gone from casual to kinky in the blink of an eye. "Well, the woman you were speaking with earlier would probably be game," she said.

"There's no sport if the prey chases you," Jeremy laughed. "Anyway, I prefer a girl who isn't so... experienced."

"I'm not a virgin," said Lily, not sure if she should be offended.

"Bet you are," he taunted, "at least for what I had in mind."

Lily held his gaze. Jeremy was handsome, and despite his sudden cockiness—or perhaps because of it—she found him appealing. He smiled temptingly, and she felt emboldened. Whatever he was proposing, why shouldn't she be game? She'd had her fill of holding up the wall at house parties. She'd always wondered what it would be like to sneak off to an empty room with a guy. It was about time she found out. She returned Jeremy's smile, accepting his dare.

He didn't waste any more time on pleasantries. "Get onto your hands and knees," he said as he undressed himself. Without giving herself time to change her mind, Lily obeyed. With his cock already rigid and standing out from his body, Jeremy knelt behind her and roughly pushed her skirt up over her ass and onto her back. He gripped the sides of her panties and pulled them down over her hips to her knees.

Lily bit her lip. In an instant, she had gone from wallflower to whore. She was on her hands and knees on the floor, presenting her naked ass to a complete stranger. Feeling her resolve breaking at the indecency, she was just about to grab for her panties when Jeremy's hands began to caress her bare buttocks. She bit her lip harder as

his palms roamed brazenly over her ass, his fingers slipping into her crack before squeezing the fleshy cheeks hard.

"You're creaming already," he muttered. "That feels good, doesn't it?"

Lily felt her nipples tighten and the friction of her bra against them sent shivers of arousal to her pussy. Jeremy's hands continued to move all over her ass, immodestly exploring and invading. The nerves on her exposed skin ignited with each of his strokes, caresses, and squeezes as the warm rush of arousal spread from her ass and pussy to her entire body. Jeremy spread her ass cheeks and ran a finger over the tight sphincter, then continued downward to her pussy, where he tickled her clit with his fingertip. Lily exhaled sharply, causing Jeremy to utter a long, low moan.

"Lean down on your elbows," Jeremy whispered. "I want your ass in the air."

Breathing heavily now, Lily lowered her chest to the floor. She was overcome by a disturbing sense of erotic vulnerability as Jeremy's hands and fingers moved more eagerly, more aggressively over her buttocks, along her crack, and against her pussy. She felt pressure against her anus and realized it was his thumb pressing against it. Her heart pounded as she realized what he was after. She muttered a pained no, but the pressure against her sphincter only intensified. And then it disappeared, followed by a jarring flare of pleasure as the tip of Jeremy's tongue touched her clit.

"Yes, you're creamy," he groaned. "You're excited by it, aren't you?" He circled her clit with the tip of his tongue, letting it dip into her pussy to lick up her wetness. Lily's hips began to move in small circles, her desire obviously overwhelming her. Jeremy pushed the tip of his tongue against her asshole, and her body writhed, forcing

him to hold on to her hips to keep her in place. He penetrated her ass with his tongue, and she shuddered long and hard. "Are you ready to lose your cherry?" he asked breathily.

Lily said nothing, but the way her hips moved so desperately made her answer clear. Holding on to the base of his erect cock, Jeremy rubbed the turgid head against Lily's pussy and spread her juices to her anus. In one motion, he sank his thick length into her pussy and began to thrust rhythmically, pushing her head and shoulders against the floor with each pump.

For the second time this evening, Lily's head was spinning. She was being fucked, wonderfully fucked, for the first time in ages. Again, she felt the unnerving pressure against her asshole and instinctively tightened the sphincter in resistance. "Relax," she heard Jeremy say. "It'll feel good if you relax." Lily focused on relaxing the muscle, and almost immediately she felt Jeremy's thumb slide past the tight ring of her anal sphincter. She was struck by an irresistible feeling of fullness. She had no idea such a feeling was even possible.

Lily was only vaguely aware of the moans coming from her own mouth. She licked her lips and tried to ignore the sudden spikes of pain that accompanied the paralyzing pleasure of Jeremy's thumb in her ass. With each thrust of his cock, he pushed his thumb deeper, further past the sphincter, until his thumb was all the way in and his hand was pressed against her ass. Lily's moans grew louder as she reveled in the idea of double penetration, in the feeling of being fucked in both places, and in the fullness. Jeremy's groans grew louder, too. He bucked hard, and Lily felt four hot bursts of liquid fill her pussy.

"Now it's your turn," Jeremy panted as he withdrew his cock. His mouth came down on Lily's ass, and again she felt his tongue

probing the sphincter, struggling to squirm past it. Jeremy slid two fingers inside her pussy and began to finger-fuck her slowly, patiently, his fingers working with his tongue to make her orgasm swell. "I want you to come," he ordered.

His tongue squeezed through Lily's sphincter and swirled around just inside her ass. Two fingers of one hand were pumping her pussy, while his other hand worked from underneath, the fingers strumming her clit. In perfect synchronicity with his finger fuck, Jeremy began to tongue-fuck Lily with the same speed and rhythm. The effect was dizzying, and Lily fought to steady herself.

Out of the rhythmic pleasure of the double penetration, Lily sensed an orgasm mounting. Its ascent was slow—frustratingly, agonizingly slow—but exquisitely steady. It peaked with an un-anticipated fury, however, and the muscles of her pussy and ass suddenly began to contract together in powerful, crippling currents of unrelenting orgasmic force. It lasted a long time, long enough that it crossed the threshold from pleasure to pain.

As her climax finally loosened its grip on her, Jeremy slowly withdrew his tongue and fingers from Lily's body. Lily collapsed onto the floor, hastily pulling her skirt back down to cover herself.

"Congratulations, you're not a wallflower anymore," said Jeremy, as he exhaustedly pulled his shirt back on.

Lily offered him a spent grin. "I'm not a virgin anymore, either."

Female Sexual Fantasy

Believe it or not, you boys aren't the only ones who have fantasies. Women have them, too. Discovering what your woman fantasizes

about and then exploiting the idea of those imaginary trysts can heighten her arousal. This doesn't need to entail a full-scale role play, complete with costume changes and a set stage (although it can, if you have the time and the resources). Whispering a sexy image or idea into your woman's ear is often enough and can really get her in the mood for love. Encourage your partner to share her lustful thoughts—share your own first, to break the ice—and then slip her fantasies into foreplay to help warm her up.

You can also use the erotic stories we've included as the foundation for a few female-friendly sex fantasies. Indulge your woman in these dreamy fantasy worlds as you perform body kissing and cunnilingus. For example, you can give your bathtub or shower a makeshift makeover by purchasing a luxurious body wash and a new loofah or sponge, and by lighting candles to mirror the erotic atmosphere in The Rendezvous. To bring the naughtiness of The Wall Flower out of the fantasy realm, lead your woman out of the bedroom, into another room: The den, garage, laundry room, closet, even the porch will do nicely.

Finally, you can make your bedroom into a spa to facilitate The Total-Body Treatment. The next chapter, The Skin-Tingling Treatment, has all the directions you need to bring this ultrasensual scenario to life.

Smile and the World Smiles with You

While this chapter suggests some great ways to help set the mood for a full-body kiss and cunnilingus, it is ultimately *your* mood that determines the sensual aura that accompanies the experience. Your

attitude is paramount. It's also infectious. If you're not enthusiastic about what you're doing, your woman will notice, and her pleasure will plummet. On the other hand, if you approach oral sex and seduction with genuine affection and eager sexual joy, her enjoyment will soar. A smile sets the sexiest mood of all, so flash your ivories, and let your woman know how happy her pleasure makes you.

4 | The Skin-Tingling Treatment

n the first chapter of *Lip Service*, we talked about the thousand daily details and distractions in a woman's life that can prevent her from experiencing sexual enjoyment. Stress is an antiaphrodisiac. It's also an epidemic. To fight this epidemic, women around the world flock to day spas, salons, and relaxing resorts, all in pursuit of soul-soothing peace. In addition to tranquillity, women visit spas to be physically pampered. The sensual beings they are, it is pure body bliss for women to receive a good foot rub, a nice body massage, and the rich sensorial indulgence of hot-stone therapy.

The four-part, skin-tingling treatment in this chapter—comprised of a foot rub, sensual massage, warm-stone caress, and erotic feathering—can both soothe and stimulate a woman's body, making it ripe and ready for the pleasures of full-body kissing. But don't fear—these practices are deceptively simple to perform. With minimal effort and prep time, you'll be a certified PPP: professional pleasure provider. To add mental eroticism to the physical pleasures of the flesh, tell your woman a sexy story while you

work. The Total-Body Treatment fantasy from the previous chapter provides ideal material for such a story.

Before you begin, transform your bedroom into a private sex spa by dimming the lights and placing a few aromatherapy candles around the room. Raise the room's temperature slightly, unplug the phone, and play some soft instrumental music. If your little darlings aren't at Grandma's, put them to sleep, and lock your bedroom door.

Part I: Foot Massage

SUPPLIES

A large basin (big enough for your partner's feet)
Two towels
Foot soak
Foot exfoliating crème or scrub
Foot moisturizing crème

You can find quality foot soaks, exfoliating scrubs, and moisturizing foot creams at almost any drugstore, although "bath-and-body" shops offer a richer selection of products, many of which contain essential oils and sea salts. If you don't have time to shop, raid your kitchen cupboards. A few tablespoons of baking soda in a basin of warm water is a nice foot soak; a paste of brown sugar or table salt and water has good exfoliating properties; olive oil is a natural moisturizer (a few drops will do; you don't want her to slip!). Follow these step-by-step moves to perform a simple yet sumptuous foot massage:

Step 1: Place a towel on the floor at the end of your bed. Fill a basin with warm water, dissolve the foot soak in the water, and set the basin on top of the towel on the floor. Place your supplies within reach.

Step 2: Ask your woman to sit on the edge of the bed and place her bare feet in the basin of water. Let her feet soak for several minutes while she rests back on her arms or lies back on the bed, perhaps on some pillows you've placed there.

Step 3: Sit or kneel at your woman's feet and lay a towel over your lap. Take one of her feet out of the basin and rub it with a small amount of exfoliating scrub, concentrating on her heel and any other rough spots. Return her foot to the basin and use the water to remove the exfoliating scrub residue.

Step 4: Repeat the above process with her other foot.

Step 5: Take both feet out of the water, towel-dry each in turn, and place them on the towel on your lap. (You won't need the water anymore, so push it aside if you wish.)

Step 6: Rub a handful of foot crème between your palms. Apply it to one foot, covering the ankle, heel, sole, arch, instep, and toes. To stimulate circulation, place her foot between your hands and rhythmically squeeze it, starting at the toes and moving toward the ankle. Change direction and squeeze back toward the toes.

Step 7: Use gliding thumb or finger strokes over the top of her foot, first stroking toward the ankle and then back toward the toes. Use the same gliding thumb or finger stroke over the bottom/sole of her foot, first stroking toward the heel and then back up toward the toes. Use your knuckles to deeply knead the sole in a back-and-forth movement. Repeat step 7 as many times and for as long as your woman wants.

Step 8: Lace your fingers between her toes, pushing your fingers through her toes to fan them apart. Repeat as many times as she wants. Pull each toe in turn (use the edge of the towel if your hands are too slippery). Set her foot down.

Step 9: Repeat steps 6 to 8 on her other foot.

Step 10: To finish, lift each foot in turn, and rotate the ankle.

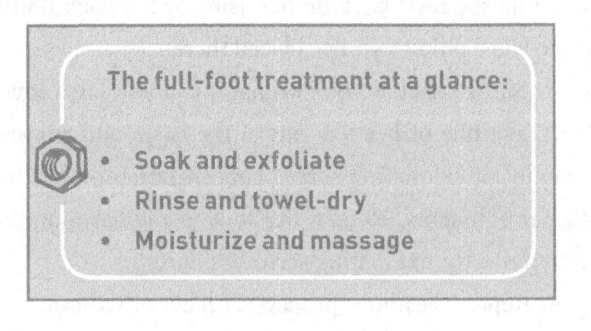

The full-foot treatment at a glance:

- Soak and exfoliate
- Rinse and towel-dry
- Moisturize and massage

Part II: Sensual Massage

SUPPLIES

Large towel or bedsheet
Two smaller towels, rolled up
Massage oil or lotion
Electric blanket or heating pad

The popular practice of sensual massage offers a paradise of products with which to bathe your woman's body in pure, unadulterated pleasure. Massage oils are available in a wide selection of scents, from nice and natural to fruity and fragrant. Different oils are also available to suit your preferences, from honey thick to

milky thin. Sensual massage creams and lotions work as well as oils, and offer as much selection. Some massage products are flavored (not always deliciously so); others have a warming sensation when rubbed into the skin, and still others pull double duty as lubes.

Sensual massage is a natural form of touch between lovers. Unlike therapeutic massage, there's no right or wrong way to caress your woman. There's only one rule: If it feels good, do it. Then do it again. That being said, it may be helpful to have an advance idea of where and how you're going to massage her. Below, you'll find a basic step-by-step sensual massage that follows a head-to-toe pattern:

Step 1: Set your electric blanket on Low (use a heating pad if you're without this necessity of northern climes), and spread an older bedsheet or large towel overtop to avoid staining it or your linen. Place your supplies within reach.

Step 2: Have your naked woman lie facedown on the bed. Place a rolled towel under her collarbones to raise her shoulders off the bed. This will enable her to rest her forehead on the bed and keep her head straight. To support her lower back, place another rolled towel under her ankles.

Step 3: Place your fingertips on your partner's head. Rake them over her scalp, along the back of her neck, down her back (one hand on each side of her spine), and over her buttocks. Beginning at her shoulders, rake down both arms, then down the back of both legs.

Step 4: Return to your partner's head. Massage her scalp as if treating her to a deep scalp-stimulating shampooing.

Step 5: Warm the massage oil between your hands. Spread it across your woman's back as well as over her neck and shoulders

in long gliding strokes. Smooth it down each arm, and then down each leg. Use generous amounts of oil, and apply it with firm but not forceful strokes.

Step 6: Knead your partner's shoulders with well-oiled hands, using the lubrication of the oil to let your hands slide all the way down her arms to her wrists. When you reach her hands, use your thumbs to stroke her palms.

Step 7: Warm more oil in your hands. With open fingers, run your flattened hands down your woman's back, on either side of her spine. Continue over her lower back, being careful not to put too much pressure on it. With your hands in the same open-fingered position, slide them up her back, again on either side of her spine. Your fingers should point the way, whether you're moving up or down her back.

Step 8: Starting at the top of her backbone, form the V shape of the peace sign with the fingers of one hand, then straddle her spine with your index and middle fingers. Move the V down and then up the sides of her spine, using as much pressure as she likes, but do not put direct pressure on the backbone itself.

Step 9: Using ample oil, place your flattened hands over her shoulder blades. Fan your hands outward in opposite directions, stroking with the heels of your hands. Move your hands down a few inches, positioning them on either side of her spine. Again, fan them outward in opposite directions, all the way across her back and over both sides. Move your hands down a few more inches, one on either side of her spine, and repeat. Continue this until you reach her lower back.

Step 10: Glide your flattened hands up her back, making circular strokes over the entire surface of her back.

Step 11: Knead her shoulders again. Use a love or lobster pinch to squeeze and lift the muscle, using as much pressure as she indicates.

Step 12: Drag your fingers down the sides of her neck. Form a stiff rake with your fingers, and rake her back downward, over her buttocks, until you reach her legs.

Step 13: Flatten your hands, and, again using the massage oil as lubrication, slide your hands down the back of both legs without using too much pressure.

Step 14: Lightly squeeze both feet as you take your hands off her body.

And now for the flip side...

Step 15: Have your woman lie on her back. Place one of the rolled towels behind her neck, the other behind her knees.

Step 16: Place your thumbs in the middle of your woman's forehead. Gently sweep outward into her hairline. Position your thumbs on the inside edges of her eyebrows, and again stroke outward from the midline. Tenderly massage her temples with your fingertips. Pull her earlobes softly. Sweep your thumbs over her cheekbones.

Step 17: Warm some massage oil between your hands. Spread it over your partner's shoulders, letting your hands glide all the way down her arms. Lift each hand in turn, first pressing your thumb into the palm and then squeezing each finger with a milking motion. Rotate each wrist in turn.

Step 18: Using more massage oil, move down your woman's chest—commenting on her lovely bare breasts, of course—and do a series of well-lubed, circular, clockwise strokes over her belly.

Step 19: Glide your hands down over her hips. Without applying too much pressure, run your flattened hands down both of her legs.

Step 20: Lightly squeeze both feet as you take your hands off her body.

Step 21: Return to your woman's head. To finish, use your fingertips to rake down her body, from head to toe, with feathery strokes.

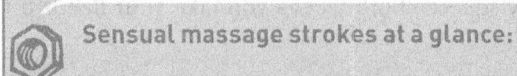

Sensual massage strokes at a glance:

- *The rake*: Over the scalp, back, buttocks, and down arms and legs
- *The glide*: Across the back and shoulders, and down arms and legs
- *The knead*: For shoulders
- *The thumb stroke*: For palms and soles
- *The V stroke*: For either side of the spine
- *The circular stroke*: For the back and belly
- *The sweep*: For the forehead and cheekbones

Part III: Warm-Stone Caress

SUPPLIES

a complete hot-stone kit or:
7 smooth basalt stones (one larger, six midsize)
massage oil

a slow cooker, or roasting pan, or casserole dish

a towel

Hot-stone therapy, sometimes called hot-stone massage or hot-rock therapy, is a healing, relaxing practice that uses water-heated basalt stones placed on key points of the body. Oiled stones are also used. If you've never had a professional hot-stone massage, you owe it to yourself—and to your woman—to book an appointment. Many fine spas offer "couple's" appointments, so forego the flowers on whatever notable event is next (whether it be a birthday, anniversary, or Valentine's Day), and double-date with a couple of massage tables instead.

A true therapeutic hot-stone massage can and should only be performed by an experienced, certified therapist, and we're not trying to offer a crash course here; however, the basic pleasures of the practice can be borrowed by couples for purely sensual enjoyment. The Warm-Stone Caress in *Lip Service* is thus inspired by hot-stone therapy. Its purpose is pleasure as opposed to therapy. The same principle holds true for massage. A therapeutic massage should be performed by a massage therapist; a sensual massage should be performed by a lover.

Hot-stone kits are available in drugstores, department stores, and online, and many provide all that you need to perform a warm-stone caress, including a selection of smooth basalt stones in different sizes, an electric warmer, tongs for removing stones from the warm water, massage oil, and instructions in the form of a video or a booklet. Some also come with a thermometer to gauge the warmth of the water.

If you don't want to invest in a kit, stop by a rock or gem shop and ask for a selection of basalt stones suitable for hot-stone

therapy. Don't let them talk you into spending hundreds of dollars for a set; several nice stones are all that you need. Choose one fairly large stone that fits comfortably in your hand: This will be your *sliding stone*. A sliding stone is the one you'll lubricate with oil and then use to stroke your woman's body. You can think of it as an extension of your hand. Also, choose six midsize *sitting stones*. Sitting stones are the ones you'll place on various parts of your woman's body and leave there, letting their warmth sink into her skin.

You'll also need some massage oil, preferably a scented one to add aromatherapy to the experience. Choose something soft, like lavender, as opposed to a strong rose. A slow cooker or even an ordinary roasting pan/casserole dish can function as an adequate heater. Fill it halfway with water, submerge the stones, and heat the water to the temperature of a very warm bath. For purposes of this caress, you'll want your stones quite warm but not hot. The water should be comfortable enough that you can retrieve and hold the stones with your bare hands rather than having to use tongs. After all, you'll be placing them directly on your lover's skin.

Follow these simple steps to give your woman a warm-stone caress:

Step 1: Place a towel under the stone heater, setting it and your supplies within reach. Your woman should still be lying on her back, basking in the afterglow of her sensual massage.

Step 2: Warm some massage oil in your hands. Spread a generous amount of it over the front and sides of your partner's legs. Hold on to the sliding stone and glide it up along the side and over the front of one leg, working from the lower calf up to the hip. Don't worry about textbook technique; use your instincts and her reactions to

plot your course and to determine the stroke/massage pressure of the sliding stone. The feel of the warm stone moving over her oiled skin will be exquisite; almost any technique will be foolproof!

Step 3: Repeat the process on the other leg.

Step 4: Spread more massage oil over the outsides and insides of your woman's arms. Grip your sliding stone and glide it over one of her palms. Glide the stone up along the inside and outside of one arm, working up toward the shoulder.

Step 5: Repeat the process on the other arm.

Step 6: Spread massage oil over your woman's chest and abdomen. Glide the sliding stone over her stomach in a clockwise direction. Glide it upward and very gently circle her breasts.

Again, for the flip side...

Step 7: Ask your woman to turn over, lie on her stomach, and raise her arms over her head (so you have good access to the sides of her body). Spread a generous amount of massage oil over the back of her legs.

Step 8: Remove the sitting stones from the heater (hold them in your hand to ensure they're not too hot), and position them along the back of her legs: Place one stone underneath each buttock, another on the back of each knee, and another on each calf.

Step 9: Glide the sliding stone up along the side of one leg, crossing over the back of the leg to weave between the stones.

Step 10: Repeat the process on the other leg.

Step 11: Apply more massage oil to your woman's buttocks and back. Place the sitting stones along her backbone, from her lower back to between her shoulder blades.

Step 12: Glide the sliding stone over her buttocks, treating each one to a clockwise massage.

Step 13: Glide the sliding stone up one side of your woman's body and then up the other. Repeat these alternating strokes several times to let her enjoy the combination of the sliding massage strokes and the penetrating warmth of the sitting stones.

Step 14: Glide the sliding stone over one of your woman's shoulders, massaging the muscles of her shoulder blade, shoulder, and neck. If the sitting stones have retained sufficient heat, you can reposition them on her shoulder area and massage around them with the sliding stone.

Step 15: Repeat the process on the other shoulder area.

Sliding-stone strokes at a glance:

- Up the front/sides of the legs
- Over the palms and up the outsides/insides of the arms
- Clockwise over belly and circling the breasts
- Up the back/sides of the legs and clockwise over the buttocks
- Up the sides of the body and over the shoulders

Part IV: Erotic Feathering

SUPPLIES

one large feather

The ultimate tingle treatment, erotic feathering will counter-act any sedating effects of the sensual massage and/or warm-stone caress, returning your woman's body and mind to a state of eager sexual anticipation.

There are two secrets to performing an arousing body-feathering session. The first is pressure: Light, lingering strokes are perfect and will result in gasps and goose-bumps. You can use either the tip of the feather to "trace" along her skin, or you can use the long side of the feather to "sweep" her skin; each type of stroke gives a deliciously distinct sensation. The second secret to perform-ing an arousing body-feathering session is placement: Find your woman's natural body contours, and follow them. For example, the mounds of her breasts and the small of her back are highly sensitive peaks and valleys that respond excitedly to erotic feathering.

Here is a no-frills feathering path you may wish to follow:

Step 1: With your woman lying facedown, arms over her head (she should already be in this position following the warm-stone caress), lightly trace the tip of the feather along the back of one leg, from the ankle to the back of the knee. Pause at the back of the knee to tease this sensitive spot with tiny feather-tip circles. Trace the feather up to just below the buttock. Use the feather's tip to trace the crease between her buttock and leg.

Step 2: Repeat the process on the other leg.

Step 3: Trace a circular, clockwise pattern on each of your woman's buttocks in turn, using just the tip of the feather and moving back and forth between buttocks. Using the long side of the feather, follow with a broad sweeping stroke to each buttock.

Step 4: Using the feather's tip, trace light, lingering lines over

the small of your woman's back. Focus on the middle of her lower back, and then travel outward to tease each of her hips.

Step 5: Begin to make your way up her back, dragging the feather's tip directly over her spine to the nape of her neck.

Step 6: Return to one hip. Using the long side of the feather, sweep the side of her body from her hip to her underarm with a broad sweeping stroke. Repeat the process on the other side of her body, alternating as many times as she likes.

Step 7: Use the feather's tip to trace along each arm, from the shoulder to the fingertips.

For the flip side...

Step 8: Ask your woman to turn over and lie on her back, preferably with her arms still overhead.

Step 9: Starting at her feet, trace the feather's tip from the tip of her toes up over her knees to the crease of her groin area (where the thigh meets the body). Repeat on the other leg, tantalizing the crease of her groin with the feather's tip.

Step 10: Using the long side of the feather, treat each leg to a broad ankle-to-crease sweeping stroke.

Step 11: With the feather's tip, trace a line up the midline of her body, starting at her pubic hair and traveling over her naval. Tickle her belly button with the tip of the feather. Keep moving up between her breasts (don't touch them yet), finishing the feather stroke at her neck. Spend several lingering moments tracing sexy designs on the front and sides of her neck with the feather's tip. Finish with a single broad sweep over her neck with the long side of the feather.

Step 12: Still using the long side of the feather and moving upward, very lightly sweep both of her sides. The sweep should start at the hip and end just below the side of the breast. Repeat this a few times to exploit this large surface area of sensitive skin.

Step 13: Using only the tip of the feather and only the lightest pressure, trace circles around her breasts in a figure-eight pattern. Circle them both, graze the sides of her breasts, and weave in between them. Tease her nipples with the tip of the feather, and then very lightly sweep over them with the long side of the feather.

Step 14: Trace the feather's tip along the inside of one arm, from the underarm to the elbow, pausing at the crease of the elbow to tease this spot. Continue along the inner forearm to the wrist and finally to the palm, ending by tracing small circles on her palm. Finish the inner arm with a single sweeping stroke from the underarm to the palm.

Step 15: Repeat along the inside of the other arm.

 Feather strokes at a glance:

- *The trace:* Use the feather's tip to stimulate "crease" areas, the back of the knees, the insides of the elbows, the spine, around the breasts, and the nipples.
- *The sweep:* Use the long side of the feather to stimulate areas you've already traced and to sweep broad stretches of skin.

Easy Does It

The four-part, skin-tingling treatment in this chapter—the foot rub, sensual massage, warm-stone caress, and erotic feathering—can work wonders when it comes to soothing and stimulating your woman. Whether you choose to practice these techniques in a single session or to spread them out, each part of the skin-tingling treatment offers a powerful way to distance your woman from her day's distractions, thereby bringing her ever closer to a heightened state of arousal.

As promised, the techniques described here are very easy to perform. We've made sure of it. For example, we know that you may not have the time (or possibly the inclination) to spend hundreds of hours (or dollars) to perfect professional hot-stone massage, and accordingly we've borrowed the spirit and sensuality of the technique and applied it to our warm-stone caress. This may fall short of a true therapeutic hot-stone massage...or will it? After all, what's more therapeutic than a lover's gentle, patient, healing touch? And no legit therapist can go under the sheets in the same special way that you can.

So don't be deceived by the relatively simple steps we've outlined for each part of the skin-tingling treatment; they have expert effects. Follow them as best you can, and you'll graduate to PPP (professional pleasure provider) status overnight. Trust us. Your woman will respect your newfound credentials more than you expect.

5 | The Art of Full-Body Kissing

See! The mountains kiss high heaven
And the waves clasp one another;
No sister flower would be forgiven
If it disdained its brother;
And the sunlight clasps the sea:
What are all these kissings worth,
If thou kiss not me?

—PERCY BYSSHE SHELLEY, *"Love's Philosophy"*

f a poem is the highest form of language, a kiss is the highest form of intimacy. Well, to a *woman* it is. The brawnier sex, however, may not always appreciate such simple sexual pleasures. Yet despite its seeming simplicity, there's no debating a kiss's strength, particularly when it comes to lovers.

When intimate partners kiss, they create and nourish the physical, emotional, and sexual bond between them. Lovers have a special inventory of kisses, from the morning good-bye peck on the cheek to the midnight kiss on the mouth. When a man kisses his woman gently on her closed eyelids, he expresses his love. When

he kisses her deeply on the mouth, he expresses his lust. The meanings of a lover's kiss are many and varied: I love you, I missed you, I need you, I forgive you, I desire you.

A full-body kiss is the ultimate lover's kiss. By rapturously encompassing every inch of a lover's body, it allows the giver to express his profound love, erotic adoration, and sexual desire for his partner, while at the same time immersing the receiver in a state of pure ecstasy. A full-body kiss is therefore a luxurious form of foreplay in preparation for both intercourse and cunnilingus. But it serves a higher purpose as well by building and maintaining a bond between lovers that no other kiss can match in either emotional intensity or physical intimacy.

The Full-Body Bond

"I knew Michael for years before we started seeing each other," explains Sara, thirty-two. "He was in my circle of friends, but not someone I knew very well. I avoided him, especially since he usually acted like an idiot. He would tell gross jokes, and when his girlfriend wasn't around, he'd talk about how she was always begging him to go down on her but how it was 'nasty' and he didn't want to. I thought he was a pig."

"Sara intimidated the hell out of me," says Michael. "She was nothing like the other girls in our crowd. She was smart and went away to vet school. When she came back, she started working at a local vet clinic, and we hardly saw her anymore."

So what brought these two unlikely lovers together?

"My dog," Michael reveals. "He'd been limping, and I took him to the vet clinic one morning when he couldn't get up. I was surprised when Sara walked into the exam room since I'd forgotten she worked there."

"His poor dog was ancient," says Sara. "He had a severe case of hip dysplasia. There was nothing we could do except put him out of his misery."

"Sara was amazing," says Michael. "I'd had Scout for fifteen years. He was an ugly dog, but I loved him. It was really hard to put him down, but Sara was great. She reassured me that I was doing the right thing, and put this whole spin on it where I felt good about doing it. I saw her in a whole new light. She was this amazing person."

"A week later, I walked into an afternoon appointment," Sara continues, "and there was Michael. He didn't have an animal with him. He had flowers. He asked me out on a date. It was very sweet... totally out of character for him."

But, as the saying goes, the path of true love never runs smooth.

"Michael was very experienced sexually," says Sara. "I wasn't. Plus, I remembered how he talked about his old girlfriend, how he hated 'going down' on her, and how he'd make fun of her. I kept wondering if he'd think the same of me."

"I thought she was frigid," Michael recalls. "It took a long time for us to get physical at all. After a while, I *really* wanted to go down on her, but she'd never let me. I talked to my sister. She gave me some advice about getting a woman in the mood, and told me to kiss Sara's whole body like it was her mouth, leaving her genitals until last."

"It was a huge change," says Sara. "Michael had never started out slowly. He'd just jump in and squeeze my breasts or something. I couldn't respond that quickly. But one night he asked me to take my clothes off, which I did, and he spent the better part of an hour just kissing my entire body. He kissed my hands, my face, my legs, my stomach, everywhere but you-know-where. When he finally did kiss me there, I was ready."

Yet it was more than just the slower pace that appealed to Sara. It was also Michael's willingness to prove how much he wanted to perform cunnilingus.

"Before, he'd just try to talk me into it," says Sara, "but talk is cheap. I watched him while he kissed my whole body. He was hard. I saw how turned on he was. He'd kiss my thigh and whisper that he wanted to kiss my pussy. It was the first time I'd seen him that excited. I needed to see it before I could really trust or believe him. To me, it was a bonding thing. It was the first time we really connected emotionally and sexually."

"It's changed our sex life," Michael finishes. "Sara's the furthest possible thing from frigid. Of all the girlfriends I've had, she's the least experienced, but she's the best lover by far. She's adventurous and confident, the perfect partner."

Sara makes an important point: Talk is cheap. If you want to perform oral sex on your woman and she's hesitant, don't try to talk her into it. Actions speak louder than words. Show her that you want to do it. Many women need to feel an emotional and physical connection to a man before they can enjoy the extreme intimacy of cunnilingus. A full-body kiss is one of the simplest, most effective ways to make this connection.

Full-Body Fun

As we've seen, a full-body kiss can help a couple build a strong bond in the bedroom. It can also bring variety and erotic anticipation back into a sex life, particularly as these often fade in longer-term love lives. Yet whatever its positive side effects on a couple's relationship and sex life as a whole may be, the full-body kiss is first and foremost a fun way for a couple to play and for a man to prep his woman for cunnilingus.

Flavored Full-Body Kissing

"I was a two-minute man," admits Jay. "Not because I couldn't help myself, but because things got stale by minute three. "We'd been together for fifteen years. I felt like I was boring her. I just did my thing and rolled off."

"Two minutes is pushing it," says Samantha, Jay's long-term partner. "Yeah, things were predictable. There was nothing we hadn't done, or at least that's what I thought. Jay was working late one night, and I watched a hot movie on satellite. The woman spread whipped cream all over her body, and the man licked it off. We had some in the fridge, so I thought, 'Why the hell not?' When he came home, I was lying in bed like a piece of apple pie. I said, 'Eat me, baby,' and he laughed."

"It was the most fun we'd had in bed in a long time," says Jay. "We hadn't done oral forever, but it all came back. Now we're

connoisseurs. She'll spread something sweet over her body—whipped cream, honey, body dust, all kinds of stuff—and I'll lick it all off before doing cunnilingus. The food's the appetizer, but she's the main course."

The Mouth as a Sexual Organ

Now that you appreciate the power and playfulness of the full-body kiss, we can turn our focus to its performance. To perfect the art of full-body kissing, a man must think of his mouth as more than just a set of lips. He must think of it as a sexual organ. Your mouth has the potential to be the sexiest part of your body. It also has the ability to elicit the strongest sexual response from your woman's body. The sound of your words, the lick of your tongue, the suck of your lips, the scratch of your teeth, even the heat of your breath are all erotic notes that you must learn to play like a master. Once a man understands that theory, he's ready to practice the art of full-body kissing.

The Three Ss: Sweet, Sinful, and Sultry

The first step in performing a full-body kiss is deciding what style of body kiss you want to carry out. While each style will arouse your woman, each also creates a unique aura that will have a distinctly different effect on her libido. Choosing the right style of body kiss and maintaining that style for the entire performance are essential if you wish to perfect the art of full-body kissing.

There are three styles from which to choose:

Sweet: The sweet style of body kissing is gentle and romantic. It can soothe your woman's troubled mind, de-stress her body, help heal emotional wounds, and strengthen the bond between you.

Sinful: This style is perfect for a night of naughty oral sex. It is best performed when your woman is feeling like a bad girl and wants you to be her bad boy.

Sultry: Passionate, slow-burning, and very seductive, the sultry style of body kissing is ideal for those evenings you want to play the skilled gigolo.

The Selection Process

Once you're familiar with the styles of full-body kisses available, how do you choose the one that's right for you and your woman? Your choice depends on many things, some of which include your and her sexual cravings, mood, level and quality of desire, life and relationship circumstance, erotic aura, sexual pattern or routine, and how much time you have to devote to the kiss.

For example, if your partner has recently suffered a loss in her life or is going through a tough time at work, you may want to ease her body and mind with a soothing balm of sweet body kisses. Sexual contact and feelings can be erotically nurturing if shared with someone you truly love. A sweet style is also perfect for make-up sex: The combination of strong emotions and tender caresses is

I love the idea of kissing my wife's body, every inch of it, but I like to see what I'm doing. Unfortunately, she makes me turn off all the lights, and I can't see a thing. What can I do to make her relax?

♀ *Debra*: Instead of turning on the fluorescents—skin doesn't look its best under them—light a single candle. Candlelight is very flattering to bare skin, and your wife might be more comfortable with that.

♂ *Don*: Good idea. After she's okay with one candle, you can move up to two. Then three, then four...

a powerful formula for forgiveness, so pull out this style the next time you're in the doghouse.

If you and your woman have just enjoyed a good XXX flick and you wish to capitalize on the heart-pounding lust flowing through her veins, you can smother her with the frenzied intensity of a sinful full-body kiss. Or, if you've just endured two hours of a romantic comedy starring a Hollywood boy toy, you can remind her of your own leading-man status by playing the role of a skilled gigolo, and giving her a night of sheet-clutching, sultry style, full-body kissing.

Variety is another consideration. Once you've introduced the full-body kiss into your love life, keep a mental note of what style(s) you've recently used. Falling back on the same style again and again will dull its impact and make the experience predictable for your

partner. Shake up the styles you use. It'll keep your partner guessing. It'll also ensure that the full-body kiss remains a potent form of foreplay in preparation for oral sex.

The Role of Role Plays

The mood you've set (see the previous chapter) is another factor to take into account when selecting your style. This is particularly so if the forces of female fantasy are at work. Recall the three erotic stories of the previous chapter as well as how these can be exploited to carry out an erotic role play.

The story line and sexual activity in the Rendezvous beg for the sweet style. The scenario of forbidden lovers finally coming together in a sexual way, no longer able to fight their desire for one another, sets the stage for an emotional erotic experience. In sharp contrast, the raw sexuality, raunchy anonymity, and taboo territory of the Wall Flower make this fantasy perfect for the sinful style. Finally, the Total-Body Treatment provides the ideal opportunity for you to show off your arsenal of mouth moves and to shower your woman with all your sultry, second-to-none sexual skill.

Stick to It

Once you've selected the style of body kiss you want to deliver, you should recognize the importance of sticking to that style for the entire performance of the kiss. This is necessary to maintain the momentum of your woman's arousal.

Imagine you're wrapped up in a great car movie. The climactic car chase is under way, and you're absorbed in the high-octane action when, suddenly, the scene changes to a slow, sentimental string of dialogue where the action hero and his long-lost lover exchange declarations of undying devotion on the raceway. Kind of knocks the wind out of your sails, doesn't it?

Changing the style of your body kiss midway through the action can similarly knock your woman's desire off course. It can also break your concentration and make your performance seem disjointed and unnatural. Therefore, make a conscious effort to stick to the style of full-body kiss you've chosen. It'll help you carry out the kiss with skill, fluency, and unbroken sexual energy. And your women won't have to deal with any poorly planned scene changes.

Kiss Classification

The French actress Mistinguette is famously quoted as saying "A kiss can be a comma, a question mark, or an exclamation point." Ah, how true, madame. The type of kiss you use on any given body part can greatly affect the way it feels to your woman. One type of kiss might give her butterflies; the next might make her moan for more; and yet another might make her gasp. Moreover, certain types of kisses are suited to certain areas of the body. A French kiss on the mouth feels rapturous; a French kiss on the ear feels ridiculous (and is probably quite deafening).

The different types of kisses you may wish to use in a full-body kiss include the following.

THE FRENCH KISS This is a deep, open-mouthed kiss in which lovers use their lips and tongues to arouse each other. A man can suck on his woman's tongue, use his tongue to circle and stroke hers, and suck on or bite her lower lip. He can also trace his tongue along the inside of her lips, perhaps passing the frenulum (the thin flap of skin that connects the upper lip to the gum) with the tip of his tongue. The French kiss is arguably the most intimate of all kisses, and for that reason there is a range of likes and dislikes. One woman may be turned on by a lover grazing her teeth with his tongue, while another may find it unpleasant. The exchange of saliva that occurs during the French kiss makes it necessary for lovers to take brief breathers and swallow, lest the kiss turn from sexy to sloppy.

THE NIBBLE This kiss is simply a gentle bite. To maximize its pleasure, try leaving your lips in contact with your lover's skin while you nibble. Areas that respond best to nibbles include the lips, earlobes, and the nipples. When nibbling her nipples, start out gently, and, if she likes it, let your nibbles get harder. Sometimes a brief flare of pain can inflame passion.

THE SUCK This kiss involves drawing an area of your woman's body into your mouth with a sexy suction action. The earlobes, nipples, lips, and tongue all respond eagerly to sucking. Sucking a woman's fingers and toes can lead to a quick wave of arousal, especially if accompanied by a whispered "I'll be sucking your clit soon."

THE TONGUE SWIRL During this kiss, a man uses the tip of his tongue to trace a small, wet circle on his woman's skin. Tongue swirls feel particularly good on the neck, the area behind the ear,

and the inner thigh. To vary the way this kiss feels to your lover, you can perform it with your lips pressed against her skin, or you can stick your tongue out of your mouth so that she only feels the tip touching her flesh.

THE LICK Anyone who's ever had an ice-cream cone knows how to perform the basics of this kiss. But there's more to the lick than polishing off a double scoop of the chocolate fudge special. By changing the strength of your licks (gentle or aggressive), the length of body surface you cover (an inch or an entire inner thigh), and the shape of your tongue (pointed or flattened), you can affect the way a lick feels to your partner.

THE BUTTERFLY For this oh-so-subtle kiss, lovers flutter their eyelashes together. Yet the eyelash flutter feels good on other areas, too, particularly those spots that sport thinner skin, such as the inner arm or the back of the knee.

THE HOT TAMALE This is a spicy kiss that can be used almost anywhere with great effect. To perform it, inhale deeply. Exhale in one long, slow, controlled breath, keeping your mouth very close to your woman's flesh, focusing your exhalation on a small area of her body. Your breath should be as hot and bothered as possible.

THE COOL FRONT This kiss is the chilly chaser to the hot tamale. The moment your hot tamale exhalation ends, pull your head back from your woman's body, and, from a distance, blow a cool breath of fresh air onto the hot spot. This is a temperature change that'll really make her shiver.

THE ESKIMO KISS Kisses don't get any cuter than this northerly nose rub. Affectionate and playful, the Eskimo kiss is a wonderful way for your and your woman's faces to be up close and personal without immediately falling into a French kiss (it's also a nice way to take a breather during a French-kissing marathon). Follow your nose rubbing with either a quick, mischievous kiss on the end of your woman's nose or a lingering, loving kiss on her forehead.

THE RIMMER The name of this kiss is derived from the sexual practice of analingus, aka rimming. Rimming is the act of stimulating a lover's anus with one's mouth, particularly with the tongue.

The way you initiate contact with your woman's anal region is up to you and her. The brave may jump in with long, steady licks over the anal sphincter, followed by confident tongue thrusts into the anus. The cautious may move slower, perhaps circling the anus with the tongue (rimming it) before cautiously pushing the tip of the tongue against the sphincter. Many women find even this slight pressure is enough to please.

Just as you can rim the anus with the tip of your tongue, so, too, can you rim other erotic orifices of your woman's body, such as the belly button, the ear flap and canal, and the mouth (specifically the surface and inside of the lips).

THE PENETRATOR This erotically invasive kiss could be called *tongue-fucking*. If performed in the anus, it's part and parcel of analingus, but, like the rimmer, the penetrator isn't limited to anal play. It can plunge its pleasure into any body orifice, including the navel (for innies, at least), the ear canal, and the mouth. If performed seductively, the penetrator can make a woman anticipate vaginal penetration.

THE FLICKER This kiss scores high marks on the flirt-and-tease scale for its quick but electrifying touch. Just as you use your fingers to quickly flip a light switch, you can use the tip of your tongue to flick over a part of your woman's body, firing up her libido. The ear canal, nipples, navel, and anus all respond eagerly to the flicker's love-'em-and-leave-'em ways.

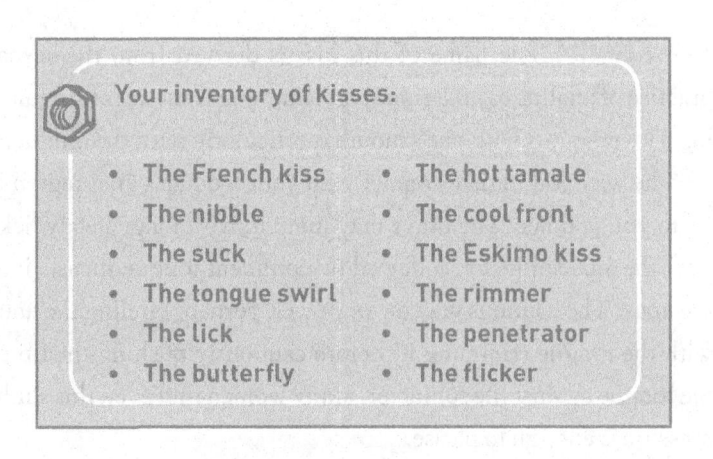

Your inventory of kisses:

- The French kiss
- The nibble
- The suck
- The tongue swirl
- The lick
- The butterfly

- The hot tamale
- The cool front
- The Eskimo kiss
- The rimmer
- The penetrator
- The flicker

The Whole Is Greater Than the Sum of Its Parts

Although a full-body kiss is comprised of a number of distinct kissing types, the whole is greater than the sum of its parts. These kisses work best when they work together. The transition from one type of kiss to another—for example, from a tongue swirl on the neck to a flicker on a nipple—should be as smooth as silk.

Practice makes perfect, and it won't take you long to gain proficiency in the art of full-body kissing. When you do, you'll find that you naturally begin to expand your skills by combining the types of kisses outlined in this chapter, thereby creating your own trademark body kisses. Such is the unlimited passion and potential of the full-body kiss.

The Three Ps: Pace, Pattern, and Pressure

The physical performance of a full-body kiss is governed by three variables: pace, pattern, and pressure. These three Ps help you carry out the style of body kiss you've chosen, be it sweet, sinful, or sultry.

PACE The pace of a full-body kiss is the speed at which it proceeds. It is determined by how quickly, or how slowly, you plant your kisses on your partner's body.

A slow pace is necessary for the sultry style of body kiss. This style is designed to be agonizingly erotic to your woman by extending the seduction phase and filling her with sexual anticipation. Accordingly, this style is perfect for the woman who needs a longer, slower warm-up phase to become aroused. The sultry style is also meant to showcase your skills as a sex master who takes his time, torturing his woman with prolonged pleasure before allowing her release. Slow kisses that lustfully but languidly travel over her body will result in an intoxicatingly sultry full-body kiss.

My girlfriend is unbelievably ticklish. If I try to kiss her back, thighs, anywhere but her lips, she just squirms. Any tips?

♂ *Don*: Tell her in advance where you're going to kiss her. It might help if she's expecting it.

♀ *Debra*: You can try to "desensitize" a ticklish spot. As Don said, let her know where you're going to kiss her. Also let her know how long the kiss will last, and ask her to try and breathe through it until the tickle lessens. Work with her to find the least-ticklish pressure: Using more pressure and then lightening up may work well. It might also help to prep the area by first stroking it with your hands or fingers, since these feel less ticklish than lips.

That being said, a slow pace can also complement the sinful style of body kiss, especially if the sexual activity in question has a fetish or taboo quality to it. For example, if your woman isn't yet at ease with anal play, you'll have to move at a slower pace if you wish to incorporate analingus or anal penetration into your sex session.

A medium pace is best for the sweet style of body kiss. The sweet style is a very emotionally charged kiss, and a medium pace allows you to perform it at a steady speed, letting your woman absorb the powerful emotions of the experience without being overwhelmed by an excruciatingly slow or exhaustingly fast pace. A medium pace

is perhaps the most natural pace to use and is therefore great for body-kiss beginners.

A fast pace suits the sinful style of body kiss. Nasty and desperate, a fast pace supports cunnilingus quickies and risqué role plays. This pace is a lusty lightening strike that hits your partner's body fast and hard. It's all about the physicality of arousal and doesn't spend a lot of time rousing emotion or loitering in foreplay. But again, sinful kisses that cross the threshold into uncharted sexual activity may have to slow down.

PATTERN Pattern is the flight path your kisses take as they move over your woman's body, landing on her flesh according to schedule. Pattern is very dependent on the position of your partner's body as well as on whether she is fully, partially, or unclothed. A good knowledge of your woman's erogenous zones is necessary to establish the most pleasurable pattern(s) your kisses should take, whether they move from head to toe, foot to forehead, or somewhere in between.

PRESSURE Pressure is the amount of force and/or compression with which your kisses fall on your lover's flesh. Changing the pressure of any given kiss or combination of kisses is a good way to increase your inventory of kissing types and to establish kissing style. For example, a feathery tongue swirl followed by a soft nibble is sweetly arousing; however, a strong tongue swirl followed by a hard nibble is sinfully ferocious. Kisses of different pressure can thus work alone and/or together to create a wealth of full-body kissing experiences for your woman.

Focusing on the three Ps of pace, pattern, and pressure will help you establish an overall flow to your full-body kiss while

simultaneously maintaining the spirit or style of kiss you've chosen. Once you learn to master these variables, you'll be one step
closer to mastering the art of full-body kissing.

> **The one, two, threes of a body kiss:**
>
> 1. Choose a style: sweet, sinful, or sultry.
> 2. Use a variety of kissing types, from the French to
>   the flicker.
> 3. Establish a flow through pace, pattern, and pressure.

Pleasure Plans

The "pleasure plan" is the final product of all your study and skill.
It is where everything you've learned about the art of full-body
kissing comes together, enabling you to devise and deliver this
ultimate prelude to cunnilingus.

Essentially, a pleasure plan is the mental flowchart you'll keep
in mind as you perform the full-body kiss. It incorporates the style
of kiss you've chosen, the types of kisses you'll use, and the pace,
pattern, and pressure with which you'll proceed. As you become
more adept at body kissing, you'll find it progressively easier to
customize pleasure plans to suit your woman's unique preferences.

To begin, however, you may find it simpler to follow the sample
schematics we've drawn up. The following pleasure plans are only
modest examples of what is possible. Play the studious pupil and

follow along to practice the art of full-body kissing; you'll graduate to master status before you know it.

PLEASURE PLAN A

Position of partner: Sitting
Style: Sweet
Pace: Medium
Pattern: Circular
Pressure: Partner's usual preference
Types of kisses used: French, nibble, Eskimo, lick, tongue swirl, rimmer, penetrator, flicker

For several reasons, Pleasure Plan A is a great one for beginners. First, it's actually a partial body kiss rather than a full one, allowing you to wade into the shallow waters of full-body kissing before jumping into the deep end. Second, it moves at a medium pace, which, as you'll remember, is the most natural and easiest pace to use. Third, the pressure you use to deliver your kisses is your partner's normal preference as opposed to dramatically soft or hard. And fourth, this body kiss is performed in the sweet style. How better to introduce this loving art into your sex life?

This partial body kiss is most easily performed if your partner is fully unclothed. Choose a night when you and she are snuggling naked under the covers, perhaps reading The Rendezvous together. To begin the body kiss, ask her to sit on the edge of the bed while you kneel on the floor between her legs. Even better, ask her to share a shower or bath with you, then sit on the edge of the tub while you stay in the warmth of the water.

Once she's comfortably seated and you're at her feet, ask her to lean over and kiss you. Meet her mouth softly, and part your lips, caressing her lips with feathery kisses and teasing nibbles before transitioning into a deeper French kiss. Gently suck her tongue and brush against it with your tongue. Remember that the very intimate nature of French-kissing makes it highly subjective. If your woman likes it, slide your tongue along the inside of her lips, lick along her teeth, suck and stroke her tongue, and explore her mouth.

Since this pleasure plan is a bonding one, don't rush through the French kiss. Instead, intersperse it with Eskimo-kiss time-outs. This gives you opportunities to swallow while maintaining the romantic aura of the body kiss. When you're ready to move on, place a line of soft kisses down the midline of your woman's body from her neck to her navel.

Because the pattern of this partial body pleasure plan is circular, it will help if you can visualize a circle whose perimeter runs through your woman's belly button, down over her hips, and across her midthighs. Her genitals are in the circle's center. Except for her genitals, which will have to wait until the chapter on cunnilingus for their share of attention, you will be kissing the area within the circle as well as the circumference.

Beginning at your woman's belly button and moving clockwise, plant a perimeter of simple kisses across her stomach. Continue the kisses down her left side and hip, over the front of both thighs, and then up her right hip and side, completing the circle at her navel. This both outlines and stimulates the area you'll be working in.

If this is a bath-time body kiss, cup some water in your hands and shower your woman's thighs, hips, and navel with it. This adds wet warmth to the feel of your mouth. Bring your mouth to her

navel and kiss it softly; then use the tip of your tongue to rim the outer edge of her belly button. Lift your head and flick each of her nipples with the tip of your tongue. Return to kissing her navel.

Following the clockwise perimeter of the circle, move to her left side with one long lick. Stop over her hip to perform one or two tongue swirls. Place a path of kisses over the front of her thigh. Treat her inner thigh to a single long lick, ending the lick in a tongue swirl near the top of her inner thigh, suggestively close to but not touching her vulva. Give her other inner thigh the same treatment.

Continue up your woman's right hip and side in a progression of long and short licks, each interrupted by tongue swirls. Don't forget

Pleasure Plan A at a glance:

- Have your woman sit as you kneel between her legs.
- Begin by French-kissing her mouth.
- Kiss down her neck to her navel.
- Place a circle of kisses across her belly, down one hip, across her thighs, and up her other hip.
- Rim her belly button.
- Flick her nipples and again kiss her navel.
- Place a circle of kisses down one hip, across her thighs, and up her other hip.
- Rim and penetrate her belly button.
- Follow the circle again, drawing ever closer to her vulva.

to moisten the trail by splashing or spreading water over her skin. When you reach her navel, use the tip of your tongue to perform another rimmer; however, follow this one by penetrating her belly button with your tongue, slowly wriggling it inside the orifice. You can whisper how you can't wait to do the same to her pussy.

Continue to follow the circle in a clockwise direction as many times as you wish, drawing closer to her vulva and letting her anticipation build. The purpose of this exercise is to increase her arousal and to subject her to delayed gratification. Don't give in to the allure of her genitals too soon! Body kissing is cunnilingus foreplay, so practice some self-restraint.

PLEASURE PLAN B

Position of partner: Supine
Style: Sultry
Pace: Slow
Pattern: Head to Toe
Pressure: Light, average, and strong
Types of kisses used: French, nibble, suck, tongue swirl, lick, butterfly, hot tamale, cool front, Eskimo, rimmer, penetrator, flicker

Pleasure Plan B is perhaps the quintessential full-body kiss. This one is a virtual cat bath that will have your woman purring with delight. To begin, have her lie naked on her back, looking up at the ceiling. This exposed position presents the best canvas on which to create this sultry-style, full-body–kiss masterpiece and to show your woman what a sexual artist you are. It's best if she's

lying in comfort on the bed, since she's in for a long session of slow-paced passion. If you're incorporating elements of The Total-Body Treatment fantasy into this posh body kiss, set an electric blanket or heating pad on medium-low, cover it with a towel or sheet, and have her lie on top.

The kissing pressure you'll use during this full-body kiss is variable: light pressure one moment, stronger the next; a hard suck or nibble on one area, then a soft suck or nibble on the next. The pattern you'll follow here is head-to-toe, but this pleasure plan can work just as well from the ground up. As long as you cover every area of your woman's body in sequence—again, with the exception of those "special spots," which are dealt with in chapter 8—you're on the right track.

Begin by simply placing a soft, welcoming kiss on your woman's forehead. Next, slowly move your face close to her and give her an intimate Eskimo kiss, letting your noses rub for several long moments before, ever so sultrily, moving your nose to her ear. Nuzzle her ear with your nose, and then, again with slow, seducing speed, breathe into her ear. Let the tip of your tongue touch her ear. Linger there before rimming the canal. Slide the tip of your tongue into her ear canal, penetrating it. A whispered "Imagine this is your pussy," won't hurt. As you withdraw your tongue, draw her earlobe into your mouth and nibble it. Transition into a tongue swirl on the area behind her earlobe.

When you're finished with that ear, brush your face against her cheek as you move your mouth to meet hers. French-kiss her gently at first, then let your mounting desire show as your kisses turn deeply desperate. Explore her mouth, suck on her tongue, suck and nibble her lower lip. Again, brush your face against hers as you

move to her other ear. Perform the same rimming, penetrating, nibbling, and tongue-swirling kisses on this ear as you did on the first.

Move at a lustful yet leisurely pace down the side of her neck, treating this ultrasensitive area to a series of light kisses, licks, and tongue swirls. Keep your lips against your woman's skin as you plant wet, eager tongue swirls, effectively French-kissing her neck. Move your kisses to the center of her neck, tongue the area, and then travel up the other side of her neck, again with a bevy of light kisses, licks, and tongue swirls.

Although your mouth is the star player in a full-body kiss, your hands are great costars. Use them in a supporting capacity by gently dragging your fingers over an area of your woman's body, stimulating her skin, and making it anxious for your mouth. Lift her arms over her head. Graze both of her inner arms with your fingertips, up and down. Lean over and give her a barely-there butterfly kiss on the inner elbow of one arm. Move to the other inner elbow and perform a hot tamale, quickly followed by a cool front. With her arms still over her head, the sides of her body—those large erogenous zones—are more accessible and more sensitive to the touch. Glide your fingertips up and down her sides, and then place soft kisses along this stretch of skin.

Next, slowly travel down your woman's chest with alternating long and short licks, some too hard, others too soft. When you reach her breasts, hold one of them in your hands and lick all around it with your flattened tongue, moving ever-inward toward the areola and nipple. Trace the areola with the tip of your tongue. Flick the nipple with your tongue, and then suck it, softly at first and then as hard as she likes. Nibble her nipple, and then experiment with a

gentle bite. Move to the other breast and repeat the process. Don't rush it; a woman's breasts and nipples can be supremely sensitive.

When you're ready to move on, plant a row of kisses down the centerline of your woman's body until you reach her navel. Remember to keep your speed in check. You might be feeling more eager, but set your libido on cruise and maintain a slow mph, even as your desire—and your woman—tempt you to pick up the pace on the downhill stretch.

Again, drag your fingertips down your woman's sides, all the way from the sides of her breasts to her hips. Retrace your steps

Pleasure Plan B at a glance:

- Have your woman lie down, and then place a welcoming kiss on her forehead.
- Kiss her ears and mouth.
- Place licks and tongue swirls on her neck.
- Graze her inner arms and the sides of her body with your fingertips.
- Place kisses on her inner elbows and the sides of her body.
- Kiss each breast: Trace the areola, then lick and suck the nipple.
- Kiss down the centerline of her body to her navel.
- Lick down to her pubic hair, and then lick over her hips.
- Place tongue swirls and nibbles on her upper inner thighs.

with soft kisses, and then move inward to her belly button in one long lick. Rim the opening and then penetrate it with your tongue. If she's an "outie," flick the button with the tip of your tongue before sucking it.

When her navel's had enough, lick downward to where her pubic hair starts. Carry the lick over her hip. As you did with her inner arms and her sides, drag your fingertips along her inner thighs to prep them for your kisses. Tongue swirls and nibbles to the inner thighs will result in a strong ache in the groin, so don't cave if she tries to coax you toward her genitals. Instead, move very close to her vulva and gently tongue the skin of her upper inner thigh.

When you're ready to wrap up this sultry full-body kiss, place a path of soft kisses down your woman's legs until you reach her feet. If she isn't ticklish, you can softly kiss her toes and suck on them.

PLEASURE PLAN C

Position of partner: Standing, then on all fours
Style: Sinful
Pace: Fast, then slow
Pattern: Head to toe, then circular
Pressure: Strong, then light
Types of kisses used: French, suck, bite, tongue swirl, lick, flicker, rimmer, penetrator

Pleasure Plan C begins as a fast-paced, aggressive body kiss with rough-and-tumble contact. It ends as a slow-paced, adventurous, slightly taboo kiss. At the start, your woman will be standing against a wall. At the end, she'll be down on all fours.

To initiate this sinful body kiss, catch your clothed woman off guard and assertively push her back against a wall. If you're following The Wall Flower fantasy, make it a wall outside the bedroom. Press your body against your woman's and give her a desperate, deep French kiss on the mouth. Bite her lower lip and suck her tongue. Clutch her clothing and struggle to slip your hands up her shirt. Take a step back and undress yourself, ordering her to do the same.

When you're both undressed, spin your woman around so that her bare breasts are pressed against the wall. You now have access to the nape of her neck, her back, her buttocks, and the backs of her legs, all areas you may normally neglect in favor of her flashier (and fleshier) frontal parts.

Attack the nape of your woman's neck with a hard, wet tongue swirl. Bite the sides of her neck and the tops of her shoulders. Quickly, drag your mouth down her spine, leaving a trail of licks and tongue swirls along the length of her backbone. As you reach her lower back, grab her hips. Bathe her lower back and then her buttocks in a frenzy of tongue swirls, licks, and bites. Continue down the back of her legs, flicking your tongue over the back of her knees.

Okay, it's time to change the pace of this body kiss from fast to slow. Why, you ask? Because this part of the pleasure plan entails a partial-body kiss that focuses on the anus. While anal play is a large part of many couples' sex lives, not all couples have ventured into this somewhat taboo territory. To make your woman's dérrière deflowering as stress free as possible, proceed slowly and with great respect. If you want your woman to remain receptive to anal play, she must know that you will stop or slow down whenever she wants.

♥ *A caveat about analingus:* It may be sexy, but it isn't always safe. At the very least, a shower is essential to ensure good anal hygiene. If there are *any* risk factors associated with you and your partner performing this activity, including but not limited to the presence or possibility of STDs, hepatitis, or intestinal parasites, use a barrier over the anus (like a dental dam, a condom that's been slit open, or even plastic food wrap) or find your fun elsewhere. If you intend to follow analingus with cunnilingus, an anal barrier *must* be used to prevent the spread of bacteria and infection. Vaginal flora is as delicate as it sounds. Once your mouth or fingers make contact with your woman's anus, her vagina is off limits until they're scrubbed to a germ-free shine.

Now that we have the warning out of the way, let's get back to the action. Urge your woman onto the floor and have her rest on all fours. Kneel behind her. Just as you worked in a circular pattern in Pleasure Plan A, so, too, will you follow a clockwise circular motion in Pleasure Plan C. Think of it as the flip side of A: When your woman is on her hands and knees in front of you, the circle arcs over her lower back, runs down one hip, arcs across the back of the upper thighs, and then runs up the other hip to return to her lower back. Her buttocks should fill most of the circle's area, and her anus should be bull's-eye center.

To begin this part of the body kiss, caress your woman's buttocks with your hands, perhaps delivering a tender love slap to her behind to get her blood flowing. Explore the area of your circle with your hands, running your palms over her hips and across the back of her legs. Knead her buttocks gently, separating them slightly to let your thumbs lightly graze her anus.

Next, kiss your woman's lower back with a soft tongue swirl

so that she can feel the warmth of your mouth on her skin. Traveling clockwise, leave a trail of soft kisses over her hip. When you reach the back of her leg, change from soft kisses to gentle tongue flicks and nibbles. Nibble and flick the tip of your tongue over the back of her other leg before kissing her other hip and returning to the starting line of her lower back. Repeat this circling-in pattern, drawing closer to her anus with each pass, until she is primed for analingus. To keep each circle fresh and exciting, change the pressure with which you perform the different types of kisses.

Separate your partner's buttocks to expose her anus. Ask her permission to kiss it. When she says yes, place soft kisses on the sphincter. Stop. Ask her if you can do more. When you have the go-ahead, kiss her anus again, then, stick your tongue out and begin to circle or rim it. Stop. Again, ask for permission to proceed, and, when you have it, lick her anus with your flattened tongue.

This initial series of kisses, rimmers, and licks should be performed at a slow pace in a reassuringly predictable pattern and with light pressure. Pause at regular intervals to tell her how turned on you are. This will increase her sexual confidence while also giving her time to absorb what is happening. Anal-region regulars may not require this kind of TLC, but newbies need it.

If your girl is game to go further, spread her buttocks apart and spend a few moments rimming her anus. Press your tongue against the sphincter, gently upping the pressure until your tongue tip slips through. Push your tongue in as far as you and/or she are comfortable with. She may enjoy the feel of your tongue wriggling around just inside her anus. She may also experience pleasure from your tongue thrusting in and out of her anus, rhythmically penetrating her. Continue kissing her as long as you or she likes.

Pleasure Plan C at a glance:

- While standing, begin with a deep, desperate French kiss on the mouth.
- Undress, and spin her around so her breasts are pressed against the wall.
- Aggressively kiss her nape, back, buttocks, and the back of her legs.
- Push her onto all fours and massage her buttocks.
- Place a circle of kisses across her lower back, over one hip, across the back of her legs, and up her other hip. Repeat, drawing ever closer to her anus.
- Lick, rim, and penetrate her sphincter with your tongue.

The Best-Laid Plans

Having a pleasure plan is essential when embarking on a full- or even partial-body kiss. Not having one is like going grocery shopping without a list: You end up wandering the aisles, wasting time, and forgetting half the items you need to buy. To get the job done with efficiency and skill, always plan your body kiss in advance. While the sample plans we've included are good teaching tools, they're not right for everyone. Even the best-laid plans sometimes need revising to avoid going awry, and we won't take it personally

if you choose to use these plans as general guidelines rather than carved-in-stone schematics.

For example, you can mix and match the types of kisses you use, or adjust the pace, pattern, and/or pressure for even more variety. You can even experiment with performing each pleasure plan in a different style. In the end, the plan is yours to lay. Full-body kissing is an art, not a science. Expand your erotic creativity and stretch your sexual imagination to keep the passion of this very special practice alive in your love life.

6 Her Parts

ave you ever heard the term *vagina dentata*? It's Latin for "toothed vagina." Send a chill up your spine? As ridiculous (and maybe misogynistic) as this concept is, it was nonetheless part of an ancient myth that reflected the male fear of female genitalia. Yet while the myth and the fear are gone, a certain ambivalence toward a woman's "parts" often still exists among modern men. We'll call it *vagina ignorata*. It's Latin for "ignorance of the vagina."

It is remarkable how many men, even very sexually experienced ones, will admit to a somewhat vague understanding of female genital anatomy. Sure, most guys are familiar with the vagina (insert A into B) and the clit (press for pleasure), but the numbers drop when they're asked about the anatomical location of the G-spot, the sensitivity of the labia minora, or the purpose of the clitoral prepuce.

Yet as important as a basic knowledge of female genital anatomy is, a good lover doesn't just memorize medical cross sections of female genitalia. Illustrations can be useful—and there are thou-

sands available online and elsewhere—but the fact is, there can be a wide variation in the appearance of a woman's genitals. Even sisters can have very different-looking genitals. (When you've finished your fantasy, please continue.) The effects of genetics, aging, childbirth, pigmentation, and a woman's state of arousal can further distinguish her genitals from the next woman's. So what's a poor boy to do if he wants to better understand his partner's parts?

A Practical Approach:
The "Find-and-Fondle" Method

The approach in *Lip Service* is personalized and practical. After you've reviewed the basics of female genitalia, as outlined below, you'll take your knowledge and use it to explore your woman's genitals, discovering each unique curve, fold, and valley that makes up the sculpture of her sex. The next time you and your woman are lying in bed, pull back the covers to admire her genitals. Tell her she's beautiful—*they're* beautiful—and that you want to learn everything about her body and what it takes to pleasure it.

To do so, you'll use our "find-and-fondle" method. As you find each structure outlined below, lightly fondle it with the tip of your finger or, if she prefers, the tip of your tongue. Ask her what kinds of sensations the stimulation gives her. As she becomes more aroused, note the changes in her genitals (for example, how her labia swell) to learn not only what turns her on but also what physical and sensorial changes occur when she is aroused.

While we've included basic female genital structures, we've chosen to exclude the study of female sexual organs (such as ova-

ries and fallopian tubes) that some other sex guides contain. Our assumption is that you're here to learn about cunnilingus, not gynecology, and we aren't interested in overwhelming you with information just to prove we can. If you're just dying to learn the whereabouts of the ischiocavernosus muscle, you can do a Google search or check out a medical book.

The Basics

If you're following the "find-and-fondle" method, you may wish to locate each of these girly gems in the order in which they're listed. This way, you'll be giving your woman time to become aroused before stimulating her most sensitive spots. Diving for her clitoris and fingering it when it's dry won't help your cause. Take your time and give each of her parts the attention it deserves.

THE MOUND OF VENUS The mound of Venus (*mons Veneris*), or pubic mound, is the fleshy mound on which your woman's pubic hair grows. Although often neglected, it can be a pleasurable spot to stimulate, particularly in the early stages of arousal. If her pubic hair is natural, run your fingers through it. If her pubic mound is bare (shaved or waxed), stroke it lightly.

THE CLEFT OF VENUS To put it simply, the cleft of Venus is your woman's "slit." It's the area at the base of the pubic mound where it divides to become the outer lips of her vulva. Some women have tissue that protrudes through the cleft (the clitoral hood and inner lips), but some don't. Both are perfectly normal.

THE VULVA This is a term that encompasses the external female genital organs including the labia (lips), clitoris, and vaginal opening, each of which is discussed in turn.

THE OUTER LIPS The outer lips, or *labia majora*, are the external lips of your woman's vulva. They are the two prominent folds that run the length of her genitals. Depending on your woman's housekeeping habits, there may be natural, trimmed, or no hair on the outer lips.

Stroking the outer lips with your fingertips, licking them with your tongue, and/or lightly sliding your penis along them are all nice moves when you're trying to stimulate your woman's genitals. Wait until your woman is at least in the beginning phases of arousal before separating the outer lips in search of more hidden treasures.

THE INNER LIPS When you separate your woman's outer lips, you'll see two thinner, hairless folds of skin. These are the highly sensitive *labia minora*, or inner lips. Once your woman is aroused and therefore sufficiently wet, you can explore these folds with your fingers or tongue.

CLITORAL HOOD The clitoral hood is the tissue that covers and protects the ultrasensitive clitoris (it's analogous to a man's foreskin) and connects it to the inner lips.

CLITORIS The star of the show, the clitoris is without a doubt the most innervated, sensitive spot on a woman's genitals or, indeed, her whole body. Most women need clitoral stimulation to reach orgasm. While some women enjoy direct stimulation of the clito-

ris, others find it too intense or even unpleasant and prefer indirect stimulation instead (indirectly pleasing the clitoris by rubbing the vulva). Overstimulating the clitoris, or stimulating it for too long, can also cause a loss of sensation.

If you find that locating the clitoris is often a challenging, even frustrating endeavor, you're not alone. If a woman's genitals are indeed "the dark continent," finding the clitoris is akin to finding the lost island of Atlantis. But what glory awaits when you finally arrive! Considering the clitoris's hidden ways, you may need to enlist your woman's services in your search. That's okay. She won't think you're clueless; she'll think you're considerate, loving, and genuinely interested in pleasuring her.

With your woman lying on her back, separate her labia. The clitoris is located below the pubic bone/mound at the top end of the vulva, nestled between the labia. The tip or *glans* of the clitoris is the only visible part of the clitoris. It resembles a bud or button, and, because it is comprised of erectile tissue, swells when sexually excited, not unlike your penis. The *shaft* of the clitoris, the part you can't see, extends internally toward the vaginal opening.

Once you've found the clitoris, you can begin to fondle it. Touch it indirectly at first by gently rubbing her vulva and labia, and concentrating on the area around the clitoris. When your woman is wet—and only when—you can proceed to softly tap, touch, graze, finger, tongue, and even suck her clitoris directly. But again, don't be surprised or discouraged if she stops you in favor of indirect stimulation. Sexual pleasure is a personal thing. Find what you're looking for, but let your woman tell you how to fondle it. Like most stars, the clitoris is gorgeous, but it's also temperamental. Only your woman knows how to keep it happy.

THE VAGINA Simply put, the vagina is the internal canal that accepts a man's erect penis during intercourse. The vagina extends from the vulva to the cervix (mouth of the uterus), and if you're worried it's too small for your girth, rest assured: If it can stretch to accommodate Junior's grand arrival, it can handle your manhood.

While the vagina is an important part of male pleasure, not all women can reach orgasm through strictly penetrative sex. As we've said, clitoral stimulation is often necessary. It's also worth noting that many women find the first couple inches of the vagina to be the most sensitive.

THE G-SPOT As if the search for the clitoris isn't enough, now you poor lads have to look for the elusive G-spot as well. That being said, there is, in our humble opinion, an inordinate amount of stress put on this crusade, with entire books being devoted to the subject. This often puts an unnecessary level of pressure on both men and women. Men can be made to feel like substandard lovers if they can't find it, while women are made to feel like they're missing out on something.

The G-spot is (purportedly) located one to two inches inside the vagina on the front, or anterior, wall. To find it, slip your index or middle finger inside your woman, turn your hand palm up, and curl your finger as if saying "come here." The area should feel slightly rougher than the surrounding vaginal wall. As with your quest for the clitoris, it is essential that you enlist your woman's help when looking for her G-spot. Her body language will let you know if you've struck gold.

It's equally important to ask your woman what feels good, once you've found this hot spot and wish to fondle it. Some women will

find gentle stroking to be exceptionally orgasmic, and there is a belief that G-spot stimulation can lead to female ejaculation. Other women will feel an urge to urinate before or while they feel pleasure (because of the proximity of the bladder), and still others will find any stimulation of the G-spot distractingly intense or even annoying.

THE PERINEUM The perineum is a short, supersensitive strip of skin that lies between the vulva and the anus. Although often forgotten, this area responds nicely to erotic contact and can add variety to the sensations your woman experiences during oral sex. Stimulation of this area can also build anticipation for anal play.

THE ANUS No, it isn't technically "genitalia," but the anus has such pleasure potential that it warrants an honorary mention. Your

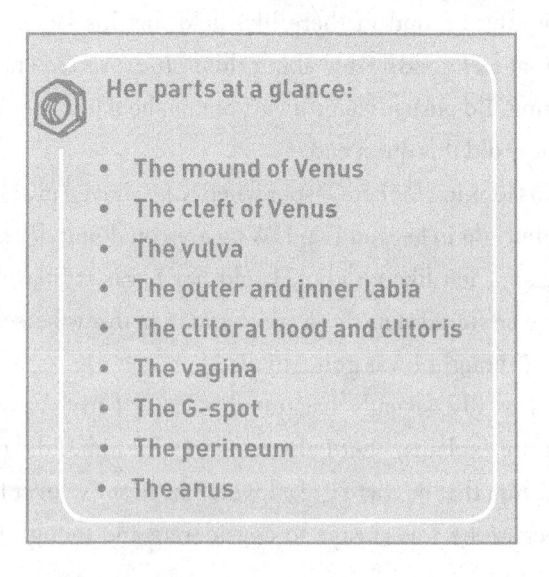

Her parts at a glance:

- The mound of Venus
- The cleft of Venus
- The vulva
- The outer and inner labia
- The clitoral hood and clitoris
- The vagina
- The G-spot
- The perineum
- The anus

woman's anal area is loaded with nerve endings, both inside and out, and anal stimulation can be an integral part of genital stimulation and oral sex.

The Quest for the Holy Grafenberg

"The article was called something like 'Extreme Orgasms: Make Her Remember You.' It was about finding a woman's G-spot." Duke, thirty-four, remembers the article well. "I had just started dating Kate. She was more experienced than me. I knew I didn't have the technique she was used to. I read that article a hundred times. It said the G-spot was the way to a woman's heart, and a guy was a disappointment in bed if he couldn't find it."

"To be honest, I wondered what the hell he was doing," admits Kate. "We'd be doing great and I'd be totally turned on, then he'd start digging around in there like he'd lost his keys. He'd ask, 'Does that feel good? How about this?' It drove me crazy. It was distracting. I'd push his hand away, but no, he'd just keep digging."

So how did this quest end?

"I was looking for her G-spot when Kate shoved my hand away, sat bolt upright in bed, and said 'Why are you doing that? Can't we just fuck?' I felt like an idiot. I told her I was trying to find her G-spot. She stared at me for a while and then threw herself back on the bed. I thought I was going to die."

"I felt really sexually frustrated because I just wanted to climax," Kate explains, "but I also felt sorry for him. I did my best to reassure him that he was a great lover. The best I've ever had, actually, because he was always so considerate and thoughtful. Duke

can use his mouth in the most wonderful ways. I love coming when he gives me oral. I've had my G-spot massaged, but it doesn't do it for me. It's hard to find, and frankly I'd rather spend the time doing other stuff than looking for it. For me, the payoff just isn't big enough."

Her Parts and Her Preferences

Just as your woman's genital appearance is unique to her, so, too, are her preferences in bed. Some women will respond strongly to G-spot stimulation while some, like Kate, get only marginal pleasure out of it. In the same way, one woman may enjoy direct clitoral stimulation, while the next can't stand it and prefers a more subtle approach instead. Your last girlfriend may have been able to reach orgasm through purely vaginal penetrative sex, but your current girlfriend may only be able to achieve climax via clitoral stimulation. Your future wife may need both clitoral and vaginal stimulation to come.

Just as your woman's genital appearance is unique to her, so, too, are her preferences in bed. As you "find and fondle" her parts, notice her reactions to your touch.

As you "find and fondle" each of your woman's genital organs, concentrate on her reactions to your touch. And keep talking. Good

sexual communication is essential to a good sex life. The male and female bodies are just too different to rely on hopeful shots in the dark or, even worse, the sensationalized sex advice pandered in glossy magazines. Always remember that identifying your woman's parts is only half the battle. Learning her preferences is what wins the day. So go ahead and get more personally acquainted with her genitalia. Despite what you may have heard, it doesn't bite.

7 | Her Passion

Women find a man's mouth sexy. Whether you are whispering sweet nothings in her ear or laying sinful kisses on her body, a woman instinctively knows the pleasure those lips of yours can provide. Good cunnilingus can give a woman the most luscious sexual sensations of all. A man's lips and tongue can manipulate a woman's genitals in ways that his penis and fingers (as enjoyable as those are!) simply can't, and many women say that the sexual joy they receive from cunnilingus is exhilarating. For some women, cunnilingus feels so good that it is the only way they can reach orgasm; for others, it is the only road to multiple orgasms.

Cunnilingus can also nourish a special sense of intimacy between partners. Like a passionate kiss on the mouth, a loving kiss on the genitals is an extremely personal act. When a woman is confident enough to present her body in such a way to her lover, she is revealing her profound trust, desire, and affection for him. And—this is what you've been waiting to hear—she'll most likely want to reciprocate.

Yet despite the physical pleasure and emotional bonding that

oral sex can create, some women still have mixed feelings about the practice. We know that many men genuinely enjoy performing cunnilingus, but there are still some women who aren't so keen about receiving. What are their reservations? Do some women just dislike it? If your woman is reluctant to receive, read this chapter twice. If she's an uninhibited eager beaver, you have our permission to skip to the next chapter.

Self-Consciousness and Cunnilingus

Even in this age of gender equality and "I am woman, hear me roar" battle cries, the modern woman can still be a self-conscious creature. Can you blame her? Every inch of a woman's body is commercialized. She's pressured to color her hair; inject her lips and surgically alter her face; augment and lift her breasts; liposuction her arms, stomach, hips, bum, and thighs; and tighten the sagging skin on her knees. And once she's achieved this perfection, she's slapped on the cover of a magazine, airbrushed to erase any last identifying features, and sold for a bargain $3.75 in the check-out aisle.

As if this isn't enough, have you heard the latest? It's called vaginal rejuvenation. It was inevitable. There's nothing left on the outside to "fix" or "youthen," so the plastic surgeons have moved inward. Now, every woman over the ripe old age of twenty-five, especially those who have actually delivered a baby the old-fashioned way, can have the fundamental feature of her womanhood sliced and diced to look like that of an eighteen-year-old porn starlet. How liberating.

This isn't meant to be a social commentary. It's meant to give men a glimpse of the relentless bodily criticism women endure every day. For those of you who are with a woman who is self-conscious about cunnilingus, you must understand her reservations before you can put them to rest.

Step into your woman's shoes. Would you feel sexually confident if the world looked at you with such a critical eye? How masculine would you feel if you were constantly being compared to the steroidal star of the latest gladiator movie? How attractive would you feel if every woman looked right past you to gawk at a billboard of a chiseled eighteen-year-old underwear model with a grapefruit-size bulge in his briefs? Perhaps you can understand why, for many women, opening themselves up to receive cunnilingus is scarier than sexy.

> If your woman is self-conscious about cunnilingus, you must understand her reservations before you can put them to rest.

Teeth, Tuna, or Tulips?

In addition to women worrying about the appearance of their genitals (Does he think they're too saggy? Am I too hairy? My inner lips protrude...does that gross him out?), women also worry about the feel of their genitals (Am I too loose?), the odor (Do I *really* smell like tuna fish?), the cleanliness (Did I use enough soap?), the flavor (Do I taste disgusting?), and her partner's comfort

(Is he tired? Am I taking too long? Am I getting too wet?). With all these worries floating around their head, it is small wonder some women can't think sexy thoughts about cunnilingus. So the question is, how does the thoughtful lover help his woman feel better about her genitals?

Metaphor is one possibility. Think back to *vagina dentata*, or the toothed vagina. Essentially, according to that myth, the vagina is a mouth—not a smiling mouth, but a killer set of jaws. That's not very flattering to the fairer sex, but happily, when it comes to the vagina, metaphor has also been used in more female-friendly ways.

The flower is a very popular metaphor for the vulva. Like a woman, a flower is soft, lovely, and fragrant. A woman's labia resemble the petals of a flower, and, like petals, her labia can open to welcome, bloom, and spread life. Comparing your woman's genitals to a flower is a wonderful way to show her that you appreciate her femininity and that you think her genitals are beautiful.

Before your next oral-sex session, buy your woman a bouquet of flowers and marvel at how the soft petals look and feel like the lips of her vulva, how the fragrance reminds you of her fresh scent, and how the nectar is like her sweet taste. As her lover, you have an incredible amount of influence over how your woman perceives her own sex and sexuality. Treat them with care and watch them

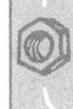

Comparing your woman's genitals to the petals of a flower is a wonderful way to make her feel feminine, beautiful, and confident.

blossom. Reassure her that she looks, feels, smells, and tastes great, and don't stop reassuring her until she believes you.

Slutty or Sexy?

Another reservation some women have about cunnilingus is that it makes them appear slutty or too sexually eager. Again, reassurance is in order. Make sure your woman knows how turned on you are by performing oral sex, and how aroused you get by watching, feeling, and hearing her reactions. Tell her that you love her, that you're eager to pleasure her in this special way, and that you want to help her explore her own sexuality. Encourage and offer, but don't pester or push. The road to reassurance may be a long one, but the destination is worth it.

Passion or Pass?

So you've addressed all the above insecurities and your woman is still uninterested in receiving cunnilingus? Is it possible that some women just don't enjoy it that much? Yes, it's possible. That may not be the right thing to say in a book featuring oral sex, but we'd be doing you a disservice to pretend otherwise. We want to help improve your sex life, not engender unwarranted feelings of inadequacy or frustration.

For many women, cunnilingus is a passionate, multiorgasmic sexual experience; for others, it's a take-it-or-leave-it kind of thing. Some women may enjoy it during foreplay but can't reach orgasm

that way. And finally, some will just want to pass entirely. It's kind of like the discussion about the G-spot: Sometimes it's mind blowing, sometimes it's just okay, and sometimes it's a no-go. Sex is a subjective game.

This wide spectrum of cunnilingus enjoyment may be a hard concept for men to grasp, particularly as receiving oral sex tops the sex list for most men. However, if your woman assures you that "It's not you, it's me," take her word for it, and don't take it personally. Regardless of what the sexperts imply, it *does not* reflect on you as a lover. Instead, put your mouth to use by concentrating on the arts of verbal seduction and full-body kissing. They can be every bit as erotic, exciting, and enjoyable.

8 | The Art of Cunnilingus

N ow that you've primed your woman with sexy talk and even sexier body kissing, you're going to secure your mouth-master status by polishing her off with some first-class cunnilingus. For those gentlemen who didn't flip ahead to this chapter, your patient study is honorable, and your efforts are about to pay off. Your woman's body, in all its glory, is one of the world's greatest wonders, and you should pride yourself for taking the time to learn about it. Not only will it make you a better lover, but it will also make you the best lover she's ever had, for a woman can feel the difference between a man who *thinks* he knows what he's doing and a man who *knows* what he's doing.

All Technique or All Talk?

"It was my first and last one-night stand," recalls Cate, thirty-three. "My boyfriend of three years had dumped me the day after

giving me an engagement ring. It sent me into this weird period of *Sex and the City* liberation. I had the engagement ring melted down and made into a nipple ring. That seemed like the liberated thing to do. I bought a leather skirt. I went hedonistic. And yes, I had a one-night stand with a guy who called himself Troy the Tongue. It wasn't my finest hour."

Troy the Tongue (a self-appointed title, incidentally) was a friend-of-a-friend acquaintance whom Cate had known for years on a casual basis. "He was good-looking, six-pack abs, the works," Cate continues. "And when he heard I was single, he was in pursuit. We had a few—hundred—drinks and he started tonguing my ear and bragging about his oral-sex techniques: He had a move called The Clitorator. Hearing him talk about it turned me on, especially since he seemed like he'd be good at it. I love oral, but my ex never did it. I was easy prey. Emphasis on *easy*."

But was Troy the Tongue as skilled as he claimed to be? Was The Clitorator really the move of Cate's dreams?

"We fooled around for a while, undressed, and he dove down on me so fast I thought he'd get the bends. I asked him to slow down, but he just gave me these really dramatic bedroom eyes. He had zero technique. I think he was just praying to the god of chance that he'd find my clit. After fifteen minutes of fumbling, he did. But he didn't know what to do with it. The Clitorator was a pipe dream. Worse, he sucked on my labia like a lollipop. I don't know how he thought that would feel good."

Tragically for Cate, Troy the Tongue was all talk and no technique. Which proves our point: Women prefer lovers who have taken the time to learn about the female form to those who just pray for divine assistance.

Cunnilingus Checklist

Before we get into the specifics of oral-sex techniques, let's look at the cunnilingus checklist. These are a few points you'll want to keep in mind at all times.

1. Practice safe sex. If you're a healthy, long-term, monogamous couple, this may simply entail cleanliness, and a barrier if analingus is part of your sex play. (Remember that an anal barrier should be used if moving from analingus to cunnilingus: If you haven't used one, clean your lips/mouth well before transitioning to cunnilingus.)

2. Give your woman the heads-up that you want to go down. A flirtatious hint will do nicely. This will give her the opportunity to clean herself up to her specs, thereby feeling confident enough to receive.

3. Think of your and your woman's comfort when choosing a position in which to perform oral sex. You don't want a neck cramp to slow you down.

4. Incorporate fingering techniques into your oral performance to compound your woman's pleasure. You can also use fingering as brief intermissions when you need a breather. Ensure that your nails are clean and trimmed.

5. Focus on keeping your jaw muscles relaxed. If your neck or mouth does get tired, stop, and ask your woman to stroke you. Let her feel how aroused you are. She'll get extra confidence, and you'll get an enjoyable break.

6. Don't make a scene if you get a hair in your mouth. Keep fingering with one hand as you discreetly fish it out with the other. Similarly, if your woman is very wet, there's nothing wrong with quickly wiping your mouth with the sheets.

7. Ask your woman what feels good, and prompt her to answer: Should I go harder or softer? Does it feel better here or here? Do you want me to put another finger inside? If she's shy and doesn't want to answer, watch her body language, and listen to her moans and sighs; they'll reveal the moves that turn her on the most.

8. When you come up for air, smile and reassure her that she tastes delicious.

9. Use what you've learned in *Lip Service*—from verbal seduction and setting the mood, to full-body kissing and skin-tingling treatments—to prep her for cunnilingus.

10. Remember that your mouth is a sex organ. Use it with skillful enthusiasm when performing oral sex, and don't let your ministrations deteriorate into a string of sloppy licks.

The Three Ss: Sweet, Sinful, and Sultry

Remember the three styles of body kisses? The same trio of styles—sweet, sinful, and sultry—applies to the performance of cunnilingus. (It may be worthwhile to flip back and review "The

My girlfriend has a strong sex drive during her period and wants me to go down on her when she has it. Is this normal? I don't really want to do it. Am I being a jerk?

♀ *Debra:* Most women would never entertain the idea of receiving oral sex during their period; however, a comparably small number don't seem to mind (some use a dental dam). But no, you're not being a jerk by not wanting to do it—frankly, I don't blame you. You should also know that menstrual blood can transmit disease, so unless you're fluid bonded, I'd advise against it.

♂ *Don:* There should be enough other things you can do to satisfy her during this time. Use a toy, let her touch herself while you suck her nipples, whatever. Women are told not to do anything they're not comfortable with. The same goes for men. If you don't want to do it, don't.

Three Ss" in chapter 5.) Each style of cunnilingus creates a unique erotic aura that will lead to a distinct oral-sex experience.

Generally speaking, a sweet style of cunnilingus fosters a soothing, romantic form of arousal; a sinful style inflames your woman's bad-girl sexuality; a sultry style makes her feel erotically indulged. When choosing a style, think about your normal approach. Is it sweet? Sultry? Whatever it is, choose the style that least resembles it to bring a surprise spark to your performance.

Once you've chosen a style, stick to it to avoid derailing your woman's accelerating arousal.

Her Wildest Dreams

When choosing the style of cunnilingus you want to perform, keep in mind any female-fantasy elements you can incorporate into the body kiss, and keep them alive as you transition into oral sex. If you're working against a deadline and have skipped the full-body foreplay, don't fear; immersing your woman in a fantasy is a good way to achieve the style of cunnilingus you want. It'll quicken her arousal, too.

Do you want to pamper your woman with the slow, sultry decadence of The Total-Body Treatment? Lay her on the bed, spread her legs, and let her lose herself in the feel of your expert mouth as it massages every inch of her body, inside and out. Or would you prefer to exploit the high emotion of The Rendezvous? Lead her into the shower, set her on the edge of the tub, and let her soak up your forbidden kisses. If you're in the mood for a raunchier role play, push her onto all fours, kneel behind her, and let her play the vulnerable, seduced wall flower.

Kiss Classification

Since cunnilingus is genital kissing, it shouldn't surprise you that the types of kisses you use will play a big part in your woman's pleasure. With only minor modifications, the full-body kisses

you learned to perform (in chapter 5) can also be used to kiss your woman's genitals. For example:

The French kiss: This deep, open-mouthed tongue kiss feels great on your woman's vulva and perineum. Pretend these hot spots are her mouth, and kiss them with the same passion.

The nibble: While as a rule you should keep your teeth clear of your partner's genitals, some women do enjoy gentle nibbles and teeth action once they're aroused. The outer labia can respond well to soft love bites, while the inner labia may like an occasional teeth graze. Go slowly to gauge your woman's pain-versus-pleasure threshold.

The suck: Various degrees of suction on your woman's inner lips and her clitoris can feel exquisite. Again, proceed with caution as each woman's level of sensitivity is different. Depending on her level of arousal, sensitivity can also differ.

The tongue swirl: This is an essential kiss for good cunnilingus. It's a rare woman who won't swoon from a tongue swirl to her aroused vulva, clitoris/clitoral hood, and perineum. You can vary the sensation of the tongue swirl by using just the fine tip of your tongue or by sticking your tongue out further and using the entire thick, fleshy organ. Tongue swirls also feel different, depending on whether or not your lips are pressed against her skin.

The lick: The lick has nearly unlimited use during oral sex. It is capable of great variety (from short and hard to long and

luxurious) and can be used anywhere on your woman's genitals. An entry-level combo is a lick to the cleft of Venus using the tip of your tongue, followed by a full-tongue lick. The intricate folds of a woman's vulva are the perfect stage for the versatile lick to work its magic, and its effect on the clitoris is nothing short of show stopping.

The butterfly: If your woman's pubic mound is bare, you can flutter your eyelashes over this sensitive skin for an ever-so-subtle sensation.

The hot tamale: Again, this kiss is a nice one for a bare pubic mound. It also feels great on the perineum.

The cool front: Immediately after serving up the hot tamale, pull your head back and cool her pubic mound or perineum with this chilly delight.

♥ *A caveat about cunnilingus: Never* blow air into your woman's vagina: To do so can cause an air embolism, a very serious condition. While neither the hot tamale nor the cool front are strong enough to knock down any walls, it's still best to restrict them to areas other than her vulva and vagina.

The Eskimo kiss: A nose nuzzle into your woman's pubic hair and vulva and against her clitoris/clitoral hood is a wonderful method of genital arousal.

The rimmer: The rimmer isn't just for analingus; rimming the vaginal opening is a guaranteed feel-good move that can make a woman crave penetration.

I love my new girlfriend, but she's "natural," and I prefer women who are trimmed. How can I get her to trim herself without sounding like an asshole?

♂ *Don:* Fashion, believe it or not, plays a big part in a guy's preference. Natural bush used to be all the rage, and the guys loved it. Now, trimmed or shaved is in fashion. In another ten years, bush could be back. Before you ask your girlfriend to change herself, ask yourself if it's that important to you. Do you really prefer a trimmed pussy, or is it just what you're used to? If it is a real preference, then you'll have to bring it up as delicately as you can.

♀ *Debra:* Trim yourself first, and then tell your girlfriend that you've heard sex feels different—better—when there's less pubic hair. You might even invite her into the shower, let her watch you trim yourself, and tell her that you've fantasized about watching her trim herself. Let her know that seeing her body in a different way would excite you. Just make sure your attitude is playful and flattering, not pressuring or critical. You can also segue into this conversation by asking her if there's anything about *your* body that she'd like to talk about, whether it's bad breath or your mustache.

The penetrator: After rimming the vaginal opening to get her juices flowing, you can penetrate it with your tongue to satisfy her cravings. Don't think this doesn't feel good because it lacks the depth your penis can reach. The vaginal opening, and the inch or so just inside the vagina are, as luck would have it, extremely sensitive areas.

The flicker: A quick flick with the tip of your tongue can spike your woman's arousal. Tease her vulva/labia, vaginal opening, clitoris/clitoral hood, perineum, and even her anus with a well-timed, well-placed tongue flick. It'll send an unexpected rush of sensation to her groin.

The Three Ps: Pace, Pattern, and Pressure

Like a full-body kiss, the physical performance of cunnilingus is affected by the three interacting variables of pace, pattern, and pressure. (Again, we recommend that you take a quick look back at "The Three Ps" in chapter 5.) The three Ps work together to enable you to perform the style of fellatio you desire, be it sweet, sinful, or sultry.

The pace of cunnilingus is the speed at which it is performed. Unlike fellatio, where a faster pace often equals a faster orgasm, the pace of cunnilingus doesn't necessarily reflect its duration. Hitting a woman with a "fast-and-hard" approach may be overstimulating and make it difficult for her to build the momentum she needs to climax.

A cunnilingus pattern is the path your genital kisses will fol-

low. It may be regular and predictable (for example, starting at the cleft and proceeding to the perineum, then repeating), or it may be unpredictable (perhaps beginning at the vaginal opening, moving to the clitoris, then to the inner lips). Yet regardless of how your mouth travels over your woman's genitals, its itinerary should be preplanned to ensure a natural flow. A good pattern can help your woman's desire build at a steady, pleasurable rate. A poor or helter-skelter pattern can distract her and detract from her pleasure.

Pressure is the amount of force you use when performing oral sex. Like pace and pattern, the amount of pressure you use to lick, kiss, and suck your woman's genitals will assist you in carrying out the different styles of cunnilingus. Varying the amount of pressure you use to deliver any type of kiss, from a lick to a rimmer, can also increase the kissing types at your disposal. For example, a soft tongue swirl and a hard tongue swirl, while classified the same, feel like two distinctly different kisses.

A final point about pressure: Many women complain that men use too much pressure during cunnilingus. It's not your fault. After

 Remember the one, two, threes of a body kiss? They're the same for cunnilingus:

1. Choose a style: sweet, sinful, or sultry.
2. Use a variety of kissing types, from the French to the flicker.
3. Establish a flow-through pace, pattern, and pressure.

all, men tend to prefer a strong suck and a firm grip. Remember that her clitoris is loaded with nerve endings, making it so ultra-sensitive that some women find direct clitoral stimulation very uncomfortable. To be safe, err on the soft side and ask her if she wants you to go harder. A flare of discomfort can be a distracting bump on the road to arousal.

Cunnilingus Contortions

The position you choose for cunnilingus is important for two reasons. First, cunnilingus takes time, and you want both parties to be comfortable. Second, different positions can add exciting physical and mental stimulation to the oral-sex experience, particularly for long-term couples. Here are a few positions you may want to try.

HER STANDING, HIM KNEELING Many men love this position, perhaps because of the novelty—chances are, it's usually your woman that's on her knees. In any case, it's a great arrangement because you can reach around to knead her buttocks, then glide your hands up to caress her breasts.

HER SITTING ON EDGE OF BED, HIM KNEELING This position lets your woman relax and spread her legs wide, giving you open access to her genitals. It's also a good angle to work from and is relatively easy on the neck. Sitting on a chair, countertop, or washing machine works just as well and gets you out of the bedroom.

HER LYING ON BACK, HIM LYING ON STOMACH This is the default position for cunnilingus. It lets your woman lie back and receive in luxury, while giving you an unobstructed view of her genitals. For variety, have her pull her legs to her chest or hook her arms around the back of her knees to hold her legs apart for you. You can also place a pillow or two under her bum to elevate her pelvis, thus relieving some of the neck strain you may feel if you're in this position for a while.

SIXTY-NINE Is it better to give than to receive? With the sixty-nine position, you can do both. There are a few contortions this couple-friendly position can sport. The classic contortion is where the man lies on his back with his woman lying on top of him, in the opposite direction, so that their faces are over each other's genitals.

To keep this classic sixty-nine position interesting, do a slow, complete roll while clasping on to your woman and still performing oral: Roll onto your sides and pleasure each other for a while, then roll again so that she's on the bottom and you're on top. Roll so that you're lying on your other side, and then finish the roll by ending up where you started, with her on top. Just be sure you start the roll on one side of the bed; you don't want to roll off the edge!

HER STRADDLING HIS FACE, HIM LYING ON BACK This position is good because it lets your woman have some control. She can lift her body if you, in your eagerness to please, happen to use too much pressure. When you're not using your fingers to part her labia or fondle her, you can hold on to her hips to urge her body

up or down, perhaps pulling her onto your face. For variety, have her sit facing your feet, then spin her around to face the other direction.

HER ON ALL FOURS You may have intercourse doggy style, but have you ever performed cunnilingus from behind? If the answer is no, you know what you're doing tonight. Have your woman get onto her hands and knees, with her bum sticking in the air. This position gives you good access to her genitals while engaging a sexy sense of nastiness. If your woman likes anal stimulation, you can finger her anus. Your other hand-and-mouth combo can simultaneously stimulate her genitals. Again, practice safe sex, and don't touch her genitals with the finger you're using on (or in) her anus.

Fast Fingers

While it's possible to perform totally hands-free cunnilingus, the nooks and crannies of a woman's genitals can make it a challenge. The following fingering techniques don't just bring extra pleasure to your woman during oral sex; they also keep her aroused while your tongue takes a time-out.

LABIAL MASSAGE Place your palm over your woman's pubic mound and gently massage it before sliding your hand down to rest on top of her vulva. Using slight pressure only, begin to massage her outer labia in small circles. Use a little more pressure to stimulate her inner labia (don't part her labia yet), and again massage in small circles. This is a good move for the early stages of sexual

contact, since it stirs her genitals without putting premature (translation: unpleasant) pressure on the clitoris.

LABIAL SPREADING Use your fingers to spread your woman's labia apart. Even the act of exposing the inner folds of her genitals can feel extremely pleasurable. It also builds sexual anticipation and makes her long for your touch.

V-STROKING Form a V for victory (peace, if you're a lover, not a fighter) with the fingers of one hand, and, holding her labia apart with your other hand, stroke up and down the inner folds of her vulva with your fingertips.

CLITORAL STIMULATION When your woman is wet—and only when—you can begin to stimulate her clitoris. Indirect stimulation is best in the beginning, so massage the clitoris/clitoral hood through the labia first. Some women won't want any direct stimulation of the clitoris. If your woman does, spread her labia and tap, stroke, or rub her clitoris. Touch it lightly at first, increasing the pressure when and if she wants you to.

FINGER PRESSURE Applying pressure to the vaginal opening can make many women eager for penetration. Press against the vaginal opening with your fingers or thumb, or curl your fingers and press with the knuckles of your index and middle fingers.

FINGER THRUSTING While some women don't need vaginal stimulation to reach orgasm during clitoris-friendly cunnilingus, others do. The feeling of fullness and the regular rhythm of a

penetrating finger (or two) can really amplify the pleasure of oral sex. Just make sure your fingers are slick with her juices or lube before sliding them in.

G-SPOTTING Once your fingers are an inch or two inside your woman's vagina, turn your hand palm up and curl your finger(s) in a "come here" motion to stroke her G-spot. Remember that some women will melt at G-spot touchdown, while others will barely notice. Even if you can't find your woman's G-spot, or you can but it doesn't do anything for her, the search can be exciting. The inside of your woman's vagina has many pleasurable areas, and G-spotting is one way to explore them. Take this opportunity to caress every inside inch of her.

I've never tried to go down on a woman. I've heard rumors that it smells and tastes bad. Does it?

♀ *Debra*: If a woman is clean and healthy, there's no reason it should smell or taste bad. Don't let rumors run, or ruin, your sex life.

♂ *Don*: Despite the locker-room horror stories you've obviously heard, many men genuinely love to go down and are proud of their oral skills. Smart guys know the favor will usually be returned. If a woman has good personal hygiene and doesn't have any health issues, the smell and taste of her genitals is usually neutral, bordering on sweet.

Oral Pleasure Plans

The oral pleasure plan is the final product of all your study and skill. It is where everything you've learned about the art of cunnilingus comes together, enabling you to plan, perform, and deliver the ultimate oral-sex experience. Similar to the pleasure plans outlined in chapter 5, oral pleasure plans are essentially mental flowcharts that you'll keep in mind as you perform cunnilingus. Each oral pleasure plan incorporates the style of cunnilingus you've chosen; the types of kisses you'll use; the pace, pattern, and pressure with which you'll proceed; and the fingering techniques you'll include.

While these oral pleasure plans are of obvious value to the cunnilingus initiate, they're also useful to the longtime practitioner whose licks and tickles have become unimaginative. In a long-term relationship, it's easy to fall back on the safety of the same old sex moves; yet even if a man has been performing cunnilingus for many years, these oral pleasure patterns will help him think outside the box...so to speak. Ultimately, an oral pleasure plan's value stems not from any secret technique or order but from its ability to motivate a man to approach cunnilingus with creativity, enthusiasm, variety, affection, and skill. Once a man can do that, he can draw up his own master plans.

ORAL PLEASURE PLAN A

Position of partner: Sitting
Style: Sweet
Pace: Medium

Pattern: Cleft to clitoris, inner labia
Pressure: Partner's usual preference
Types of kisses used: Tongue swirl, lick, suck, flicker
Fingering techniques: Labial massage, labial spreading,
    V-stroking, clitoral stimulation

To begin Oral Pleasure Plan A, have your naked partner sit on the edge of the bed with her legs wide apart. Or, share a shower and then ask her to sit on the edge of the tub while you stay immersed in the water, mirroring the eroticism of "the Rendezvous" fantasy. If you've just performed the body kiss featured in Pleasure Plan A (from chapter 5), your woman will already be prepped and in place for cunnilingus.

If you are performing this oral pleasure plan in the bathtub, you can initiate genital contact by cleaning her genitals. Not only is this an erotic way to awaken her arousal, but the assurance of cleanliness will also give both of you sexual confidence.

Make your first genital kiss an affectionate one by placing a loving tongue swirl on her cleft, letting your tongue dip into the furrow as it swirls around. Next, massage your woman's outer labia in small circles with your fingers. Massage gently at first, and then increase the pressure to stimulate her clitoris through her labia.

Spread her labia apart. Place a few feathery tongue swirls along her inner labia, avoiding the clitoris. Lick her inner labia, tracing the folds with the tip of your tongue. Continue licking until she is wet.

Still spreading her open, perform several V strokes along her inner labia with your fingertips. Only do this when she is well-lubricated. If you're in the tub, you can hasten the process by dipping your fingers in the warm water and moistening her.

Close her outer labia and massage them to indirectly stimulate her clitoris. Place another tongue swirl on the cleft, this time using more pressure. Read her body language. If she's very aroused, spread her outer labia open again, and flick the tip of your tongue over her clitoris or clitoral hood. Follow with short licks along her inner labia.

Apply a tiny tongue swirl at the area of the opened cleft. Place another small tongue swirl over the clitoris, circling it with the tip of your tongue. Suck gently. Stop sucking, and finger her clit. Tap and then stroke it lightly with your fingertip.

Close her outer labia and massage it.

When you want to continue, spread her open yet again and place one tongue swirl at the opened cleft, another on her clitoris.

Oral Pleasure Plan A at a glance:

- Have your woman sit with her legs open.
- Kiss her cleft, dipping your tongue into the furrow.
- Massage her outer labia to stimulate her clitoris.
- Spread her outer labia to kiss and V-stroke her inner labia.
- Close her outer labia and kiss her cleft.
- Spread her outer labia to kiss her clitoris and inner labia.
- Bring her to orgasm by kissing/sucking her clitoris.
- To delay orgasm, "tap" her clitoris or halt clitoral stimulation.

Flick your tongue over her clit. Lick the area around it. Tongue-flick her clitoris again, and then suck gently.

If you want to delay her orgasm, halt clitoral stimulation and return to V-stroking her inner labia. You can keep her arousal peaked without pushing her over the edge of orgasm by placing soft fingertip taps on her clitoris. As you do, look into her eyes so that she can see your desire. Strong emotions can intensify sexual feelings, so exploit the emotional charge of this sweet-style scenario.

If you're performing this oral pleasure plan in the bathtub, fill a cup with water, and, holding her labia apart, pour warm water over her exposed genitalia. A removable showerhead can also provide a great aquatic genital massage. Squeezing the water out of a soaked facecloth and dribbling it down over her will also feel good. You can also lay the wet facecloth over her exposed genitals and very softly slap them with your hand to give your woman a sensation she may not have felt before.

When you want your woman to come, focus your attention on her clitoris. Place a tongue swirl over it, flick it, and then suck until she climaxes.

ORAL PLEASURE PLAN B

Position of partner: Supine
Style: Sultry
Pace: Slow
Pattern: Pubic mound to perineum
Pressure: Slight to strong
Types of kisses used: Eskimo kiss, lick, tongue swirl, French
    kiss, flicker, rimmer, penetrator, hot tamale, cool front, suck

Fingering techniques: Labial massage, labial spreading, V-stroking, clitoral stimulation, finger pressure, finger thrusting, G-spotting

Oral Pleasure Plan B is cunnilingus at its finest. This plan lets you show off all your oral skills while bathing your woman's body in the most luxurious sexual ecstasy imaginable. This is the cunnilingus experience she's fantasized about.

To begin, have your woman lie naked on her back, preferably in the comfort and warmth of your bed. If you've just performed the full-body kiss featured in Pleasure Plan B (from chapter 5), your woman will already be prepped and in place for cunnilingus in the sexy spirit of The Total-Body Treatment.

As you carry out this Oral Pleasure Plan, keep your speed in check and remember, even as your and your woman's desires mount, this plan is best performed at a slow, steady pace. Designed in the sultry style, it is the perfect plan to showcase your oral sex skills, so don't rush the process. (Remember that you can place a pillow or firm cushion under her bum to elevate her pelvis, thus making her genitals more accessible to you and mitigating your neck strain.) The pressure you'll use to deliver your kisses, sucks, licks, and so forth will vary, although, generally speaking, they will proceed from slight in the early stages of arousal to stronger as your partner nears orgasm.

To begin genital contact, nuzzle your nose into your woman's pubic hair, introducing yourself with an Eskimo kiss. Next, place your hand on her pubic mound and press down slightly while simultaneously pushing forward (toward her head). This puts a pleasing pressure on this erogenous spot and also "raises" her

genitals somewhat, generating a feeling that many women enjoy. With her genitals in this position, slide your tongue into her cleft to lick with small up-and-down movements.

Moving very slowly, extend the lick downward, just barely grazing over her clitoris and vaginal opening, to arrive at her perineum. Place a lazy tongue swirl on her perineum, following it with a long-lasting French kiss.

Press your hand or fingers/thumbs against your woman's outer labia, and massage them to indirectly stimulate her clitoris. Spread her labia. Flick your tongue over her clitoris or clitoral hood for a few brief moments. When she's moist, V-stroke her inner labia with your fingertips to stimulate these sensitive lips, while letting her clitoris cool down.

When you're ready to heat things up again, spread her labia further apart, and place a tongue swirl over her clitoris. Apply gentle pressure to her clitoris by lightly fingering it. Follow with another tongue swirl. Read your woman's body language. When clitoral stimulation seems to be overwhelming her, stop, and turn your attention to her vaginal opening.

Rim the vaginal opening with your tongue, teasing her with every circle and making her long to feel it slip inside. Make her wait at least several moments before penetrating her vagina with your tongue. Don't worry about doing anything fancy. Simply thrust it in and out a few times.

Stop tonguing her. To continue stimulating the vaginal opening, curl your fingers, and press your knuckles against the opening. The pressure should be steady at first and then pulsating. Again, read her body language. When she's eager for more, slowly slide the length of your middle finger into her vagina.

As you thrust with your middle finger, bring your mouth close to her body and tongue her clitoris. Do this for only a short time; you don't want her to climax too soon.

Once you stop this thrusting-and-tonguing action, you can start G-spotting. Turn your hand palm up and curl your middle finger in a "come here" motion to stroke her G-spot. If you find it and it pleases her, great. Stroke it for a while longer. If you don't

Oral Pleasure Plan B at a glance:

- Have your woman lie on her back.
- Apply pressure to her pubic mound.
- Lick her cleft, clitoris, and vaginal opening.
- Tongue-swirl and French-kiss her perineum.
- Spread her labia to flick her clitoris.
- V-stroke her inner labia to let her clitoris cool down.
- Finger and kiss her clitoris with a tongue swirl.
- Rim and penetrate her vaginal opening with your tongue.
- Penetrate her with your finger and stimulate her G-spot.
- Slide your tongue into her cleft, then lick and suck her clitoris.
- Slide your hands up, to pinch her nipples.
- Penetrate her with your finger(s) and thrust.
- Bring her to climax by kissing/sucking her clitoris and finger-thrusting.

find her G-spot or she doesn't care for the feeling, forget it. Focus instead on exploring the inside of her vagina. The vaginal walls have many areas of sensitivity that, when discovered, can create highly pleasurable sensations. Your woman may not even know what she's been missing! If you wish, you can combine G-spotting with clitoral stimulation, whether by finger or tongue.

To extend the experience and to further vary sensation, withdraw your finger from your woman's vagina, and, as you do so, place another French kiss on her perineum. Follow it with a hot tamale, and then with a cool front. Finish pleasuring her perineum with a few tongue swirls.

Return to your woman's pubic mound and place a simple kiss on it. Slide your tongue between her cleft, to her clitoris, and circle the bud with small licks. Introduce soft suction into your tonguing. As you tongue and suck her clitoris, slide your hands up her body to pinch her nipples. Stimulating these three "buds" simultaneously is exquisitely pleasurable—and highly orgasmic—for many women. Spend some time doing this, as you're now gearing her up for climax.

Spread your woman's labia apart, and, still tonguing and sucking her clit, slide one or two fingers (depending on her preference) into her vagina. Begin to thrust slowly, only slightly increasing your speed as her arousal swells. Keep tonguing and sucking her clitoris and thrusting your finger(s) into her vagina, making sure to maintain the pace, pattern, and pressure she responds to best as her orgasm builds and she climaxes. If the rhythm you're using is working, don't change it last moment to help her "get there." She'll get there faster if you don't interrupt her momentum.

ORAL PLEASURE PLAN C

Position of partner: On all fours
Style: Sinful
Pace: Partner's preference
Pattern: Circular
Pressure: Partner's preference
Types of kisses used: Lick, tongue swirl, nibble, rimmer,
    penetrator
Fingering techniques: Labial massage, labial spreading, clitoral
    stimulation, finger pressure, finger thrusting

The cunnilingus in Oral Pleasure Plan C is ideally suited to
follow the body kiss in Pleasure Plan C (again, from chapter 5). In
fact, we'll be picking up where we left off: Your naked woman is
on all fours, her bum is in the air, and you're kneeling behind her,
performing analingus à la Wallflower. You may wish to review the
analingus advice and caveat from Pleasure Plan C before reading
on, especially if you or your partner are new to the practice.

Hold your woman's buttocks apart as you lick her anus with a
series of short strokes (using the tip of your tongue) and longer strokes
(using your flattened tongue). Follow these licks with a tongue swirl
to the anus. Give her a few gentle nibbles along the inside fleshy
parts of her buttocks to keep the sinful spirit of this plan alive.

Use your tongue to rim her anus several times in slow circles.
Hold the tip of your tongue against her anus, and, if she likes the
sensation, penetrate it. Begin to thrust. Whether you penetrate and
thrust into your woman's anus with your tongue or just rim the

Oral Pleasure Plan C at a glance:

- Have your woman get on all fours.
- Hold her buttocks apart: Kiss her anus with licks and tongue swirls.
- Rim and/or penetrate the sphincter with your tongue.
- Stimulate her clitoris and penetrate her vagina with your finger(s).
- Bring her to orgasm by kissing her anus while fingering her clitoris and vagina.

sphincter wholly depends on your partner. Watch her reactions. If she moans with pleasure as you penetrate, you're good to go; if she pulls away, stick to rimming.

As your tongue continues to stimulate her anus, reach underneath her body to massage her labia. When she moistens, separate her outer labia. Gently graze her inner labia and clitoris with your fingers. Continue until she is in a state of intense arousal.

Press your fingers against the vaginal opening, applying pressure to it without letting your fingers actually penetrate. When she's desperate for more, slide a finger or two inside her vagina. Rest there for a moment. Begin to thrust, finding a rhythm that pleases her. Use the fingers of your other hand to stimulate her clitoris.

Continue to tongue your woman's anus as your fingers thrust into her vagina and stimulate her clitoris. This sinful combo will result in a climax to remember.

An Alternate Ending

Oral Pleasure Plan C has an alternate ending. Instead of using both hands to stimulate your woman's genitals, you can use the fingers of one hand to penetrate and pleasure her genitals, while the thumb or index finger of your other hand penetrates her anus. Tonguing the anal area as you finger-thrust into her anus adds extra sensation.

This ending gives your woman the experience of double penetration: She has a finger (or two) in her vagina as well as a finger in her anus. It may be challenging for you to use the same hand to penetrate her vagina and stimulate her clitoris, but it can be done. For example, you can penetrate her vagina with your thumb and stroke her clitoris with your fingers, or you can penetrate with your fingers and stroke her clitoris between thrusts.

If you still want to devote one hand entirely to your woman's clitoral pleasure, however, you can use the same hand to penetrate her anus and vagina. To do so, slide your thumb into her anus and your index and/or middle finger into her vagina. Whatever way you make it happen, the feeling of double penetration combined with clitoral stimulation will be highly orgasmic.

💛 *As with everything anal*, a caveat applies. You'll need lots of lubrication to slide your finger/thumb into your woman's anus. Her juices probably won't be enough. Have a bottle of good, thick lube nearby if you plan on anal play. Also, be careful to keep your "anus" finger away from your woman's genitals to avoid spreading germs. If you're going to finger-thrust both openings barrier free, always make sure that your left hand

knows what your right hand is doing, and, obviously, don't tongue her genitals after tonguing her anus.

Plan Revisions

While *Lip Service* offers some great oral pleasure plans, you should always watch your woman's body language and revise our plans as needed to make sure you're doing what she likes.

For example, direct clitoral contact may be too much for your woman. In that case, replace it with indirect stimulation such as tonguing the clitoral hood, the area around the clitoris, or just stimulating the clitoris through the labia. Similarly, not all women will like clitoral suction. You can substitute tongue swirls or licks for sucks.

Anal play, such as that in Oral Pleasure Plan C is, obviously, not for everyone. Some women will be totally into it, others may entertain it to some degree—perhaps just letting you apply gentle finger pressure to the anus during cunnilingus—while still others will reject any type of anal contact whatsoever.

As we've said, sex is a subjective game, and you'll have to play by your woman's rules. Read and reread these oral pleasure plans to get started, but always revise them to suit your woman's unique preferences and pleasures.

9 | Girly Gadgets

A man's mouth may be a powerful sex organ, but that doesn't mean it has to play solo when performing oral sex. Female-friendly erotic aides can play along to make even more beautiful music. New World sex-toy technology can consign Old World cunnilingus to the history books. So stock up on batteries, and get ready to give your woman an updated buzz in the bedroom.

The Classics

A woman's genitals are pleasured through a combination of clitoral stimulation and vaginal penetration, and the classic female sex toys—those being the vibrator and the dildo—are as efficient in this regard as they are enduring. The modern woman, however, demands more variety than an ultrautilitarian, standard-issue, straight vibrator or a novelty-ish, vein-bulging rubber dildo. Happily, the law of supply and demand has come to her rescue. She asked for more to choose from, and she got it . . . in abundance.

Nouveau Erotica

The availability, variety, selection, quality, and appearance of today's sex toys are astounding, and a person can't be faulted for feeling a little intimidated. There are jellied tickling dolphins, buzzing rabbit ears, and fluttering butterfly wings. It makes one wonder if any member of the animal world is safe from erotic-aide mimicry. There are red spiraling love wands, hot-pink teasers, and purple remote-control eggs, proving that even the color spectrum isn't exempt from sex-toy exploitation. The sex-toy industry is expanding every day. And why not? The bedroom is big business.

Yet despite the remarkable differences in then-versus-now appearance and the lofty claims of toy manufacturers, modern sex toys perform the same fundamental services as the classics: to tickle and thrust. Clitoral stimulation and vaginal penetration are still what it's all about. After all, it's just the sex toys that have changed; the female body has stayed the same. That tickling dolphin and fluttering butterfly wing do the same thing as the straight vibrator, albeit with more flair. And that red spiraling love wand? It's an updated version of the dildo.

Our point is this: Don't be intimidated when you set out to purchase a new sex toy for your woman, and don't be influenced by the flashy colors, whirring parts, and bizarre shapes. Before you shop, ask yourself these questions: What turns my woman on the most—clitoral stimulation, vaginal penetration/thrusting, or a combination of both? When you have the answer, look for a toy that provides that service and buy it rather than the "pretty" or "high-tech" toy.

Focus on the item's *function* rather than its appearance, advertising, or cutesy name, and your sex-toy shopping will be a success.

 When buying a sex toy for your lady, think about what turns her on—clitoral stimulation, vaginal penetration, or both?—and look for a toy that performs that function.

Here are few mentionable unmentionables.

BUNNY RABBIT VIBRATOR Okay, this girly gadget has it all: dual functional clitoral stimulation (thanks to tickling bunny ears), vaginal penetration (courtesy of an updated straight vibrator), and a cutesy name to boot. How cheeky. The straight vibrator part of this toy varies by model: Some turn around; some stimulate the G-spot; and some even pump up and down. Since this toy provides a lot of sensation, you may want to use it to bring your woman to orgasm after you're finished using your mouth.

TONGUE VIBRATOR To clarify, this vibrator is in the shape of a tongue; it doesn't actually go *on* your tongue. The biggest strength of this little gem is its fine-motor skills, since the tongue tip is capable of very refined stimulation. Hold on to the tongue vibrator and use it simultaneously with your own tongue, licking your woman's labia and clitoris to let her experience the sinful sensations of two-tongue cunnilingus.

FINGERTIP VIBRATOR As with all sex toys, fingertip vibrators come in a range of models. Some slip over one fingertip, while others adorn all five. Just to keep things interesting, have your woman wear the vibrator on her finger(s), and encourage her to touch herself while you perform cunnilingus. Be sure that her genitals are wet with your saliva or her juices so that the vibrating fingertips can glide easily over/into her folds.

BULLET/EGG VIBRATOR Bullet or egg vibrators typically slide inside a woman's vagina, where they vibrate, thus pleasuring the inside of the vagina. Choose a model that promises quiet performance and multiple levels of vibration. In the tradition of your sex, you'll be happy to know that many of these come with remote controls. Slip the egg or bullet inside your woman and tongue her genitals for a few moments before turning on the vibration. Let her choose the speed/type of vibration she likes, and then continue with cunnilingus as the vibrator stimulates her vagina.

UPDATED DILDOS Remember that novelty-ish, vein-bulging, rubbery dildo we mentioned? Today's version is almost unrecognizable. Available in an array of colors, textures, materials, designs, and sizes, and boasting a range of features, the modern dildo is a work of functional art. At the very least, the one you choose for your woman should have suction cups for hands-free fun, and should be capable of bending somewhat. A highly textured surface is also a plus. Thrust the dildo into your woman's vagina as you tongue her clitoris to give her the best of both worlds.

PLEASURE BALLS Ben Wa balls have been used for ages (literally) to strengthen the vaginal muscles. They feel good, too. If your woman enjoys the feeling of vaginal fullness, pleasure balls are the perfect choice. Slip them inside her vagina and leave them in place as you perform cunnilingus. To triple her pleasure, use a dildo or vibrator to stimulate the vaginal opening as you tongue her: This lets her enjoy your tongue on her clitoris, the balls in her vagina, and the dildo or vibrator stimulating her vaginal opening.

NIPPLE CLAMPS Stimulating nipple clamps aren't just for rough sex or BDSM (Bondage, Domination and Submission, Sadism, and Masochism). The fact is, pinching or otherwise pleasuring the nipples can increase clitoral sensation for many women. If your woman hasn't worn nipple clamps before, stay away from the leather-tasseled chains and tight roach clips. Instead, choose light-weight, adjustable clamps. Place them on your woman's nipples and then tongue her clitoris. If this toy sounds too industrial for your woman, try a nipple-stimulating gel or lotion instead.

Clitoral Chic

Many sex toys include an extension or feature for clitoral stimulation (like rabbit-type vibrators), but there are also many toys that are designed exclusively for clitoral pleasure.

STRAP-ON CLITORAL VIBRATOR These small vibrators are often attached to a panty that holds the vibrator in place against the clitoris. Choose a crotch-free model that will allow you to lick and tongue her vagina alongside the vibrator's clitoral pulsations.

CLITORAL PUMP In addition to stimulating the clitoris via vibration, these pumps "suck" the clitoris to compound a woman's pleasure. You can use a clitoral pump before or during cunnilingus, but remember that some toys—particularly those without good speed selection—can overstimulate a woman's genitals. Use this pump slowly and in short increments, at least until she gets the feel of it, and don't take it personally if your mouth doesn't have the same battery power.

CLITORAL CREAM Clitoris-stimulating creams, gels, and lotions abound in sex shops. But because all women are different, results vary. While some taste fine, others aren't so palatable. Everyone's taste is different. Apply the cream directly to the clitoris, but use your tongue elsewhere until you see how your woman reacts. Again, overstimulating her genitals is as bad as understimulating them.

High-Class Glass

For the discriminating woman, glass sex toys are the ultimate in sexual sophistication. Glass toys—whether dildos, butt plugs, or double dongs—can be strikingly beautiful in color and design. But they're more than just good looking; they're smart, too. Glass toys are easy to clean, long-lasting, and boast a nonporous surface that feels like nothing else. They can also be warmed or cooled to add to the unique sensation that only glass can give.

If your woman is reluctant to bring sex toys into the bedroom,

> If your woman is hesitant to play with sex toys, try gifting her with an attractive glass toy.

gifting her with a basic straight glass wand may be a great way to introduce toys into your love life. Choose her favorite color, wrap it up pretty, and present it with a bouquet of flowers in complementary colors. If your woman can see the classy side of sex toys, she might be more game to play along.

Anal Accessories

When it comes to sex toys, no territory has gone unexplored or unexploited. Anal sex toys also abound and, like all other types of erotic accoutrements, shine in their selection. Anal beads (graduated from small to largest are best), butt plugs, dildos, dongs, wands, and vibrators are the most popular anal toys.

The type of toy you choose will depend on the type of activity you want to engage in. Do you want to penetrate the anus fully, partially, or just apply pressure to the sphincter? Discuss with your woman what she is willing to try, and then choose the appropriate toy. For example, a dildo with a smooth, bulbous tip will work well if you want to simply apply pressure to the sphincter. The tip of a vibrator held against the anus can add flair to this feeling. A thin, textured anal probe may be better if you want to go a little deeper.

In addition to pleasuring the anal area, anal toys are valuable for health reasons. If you and your woman enjoy anal play during sex, it's a great idea to reserve certain toys for the anal region only. This way, you never have to worry about germ transfer.

A final plug (no pun intended) for anal toys: If your woman has been resistant to analingus or anal play during cunnilingus, an anal sex toy could lower that resistance. Many women would never let a man use his mouth on her anus: Will it smell? Does it taste bad? Is he grossed out? Again, there's no room for sexy thoughts with those questions floating around her head. Using an anal toy may alleviate her fears while still providing the pleasure she's been secretly craving.

Slippery Sex

Lubrication is also something to consider when using a sex toy, including anal toys. For example, you'll need a thick anal lube if you're planning on anal penetration with a toy. Make certain the toy and the personal lubricant are compatible by diligently researching or reading the labels of any products you purchase, and/or by checking with the salesperson.

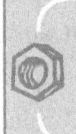 Always ensure that your sex toys and your personal lubricants are compatible.

Generally speaking, water-based lubes are best and are compatible with most sex toys, whether they're made of latex or silicone. Silicone-based lubes, while great for water play, will break down silicone toys. Oil- and petroleum-based lubes will destroy latex—they'll stain your sheets, too!

10 | Customized Cunnilingus

Even the finest designer gown needs the attention of a seamstress before it can flawlessly flatter a woman's figure. The same goes for oral sex: Even if a man has learned to skillfully use his mouth as a sexual organ and has thus mastered the art of cunnilingus, he must still customize his technique to pleasure his partner's unique body. Customized cunnilingus requires two things: practice and communication. The practice part is easy. For many couples, sexual communication is more difficult.

 When it comes to talking about sex, is your partner the silent type? If so, use these questions to pry her unspoken passions out of her. If she's the talkative type, these questions can reveal even more about her sexual desires.

If you and your woman have trouble speaking openly about your sexual desires, ask her to read the following questions in private and to write down her answers. Encourage her to elaborate as much as possible on each response. She can add new ideas whenever she wishes, thereby using this book as a communication medium until you learn to speak together more comfortably about sex. If you and your woman are already at ease talking about your sex life, you can use these questions as catalysts to explore her desires even deeper.

1. Do you prefer cunnilingus as foreplay, the featured sex act, or both?
2. What are your favorite positions in which to receive cunnilingus?
3. Do you like it when I talk dirty before and during oral sex?
4. What are the most sensitive spots on your genitals?
5. Do you like direct or indirect clitoral stimulation?
6. Do you like to have your vagina penetrated with a toy/finger during oral sex?
7. What kinds of sex toys do you like or want to try?
8. What fantasy elements would you like to play with during oral sex?
9. Do you have any reservations about receiving cunnilingus?
10. Do you enjoy anal stimulation during cunnilingus?